ABUSED MEN

The Hidden Side of Domestic Violence

SECOND EDITION

PHILIP W. COOK

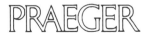

Westport, Connecticut
London

Library of Congress Cataloging-in-Publication Data

Cook, Philip W., 1948–
   Abused men : the hidden side of domestic violence / Philip W. Cook.—2nd ed.
      p. cm.
   Includes bibliographical references and index.
   ISBN 978-0-313-35618-6 (alk. paper) — ISBN 978-0-313-35671-1 (pbk. :
alk. paper)
  1. Abused men—United States.   2. Abused husbands—United
States.   3. Abusive women—United States.   4. Family violence—United
States.   I. Title.
HV6626.2.C65   2009
362.82′92—dc22   2008042616

British Library Cataloguing in Publication Data is available.

Library of Congress Catalog Card Number: 2008042616
ISBN: 978-0-313-35618-6
     978-0-313-35671-1 (pbk.)

First published in 2009

Praeger Publishers, 88 Post Road West, Westport, CT 06881
An imprint of Greenwood Publishing Group, Inc.
www.praeger.com

Printed in the United States of America

The paper used in this book complies with the
Permanent Paper Standard issued by the National
Information Standards Organization (Z39.48–1984).

10 9 8 7 6 5 4 3 2 1

Copyright Acknowledgments

The author and publisher gratefully acknowledge permission for use of the following material:

Portions of Chapter 5 in this volume originally appeared in *Family Interventions in Domestic Violence: A Handbook of Gender-Inclusive Theory and Treatment*, edited by John Hamel and Tonia Nicholls, pp. 601–619. Coauthors of the article were Cathy Young, Philip Cook, Sheila Smith, Jack Turtletaub, and Lonnie Hazelwood. New York: Springer, 2007.

Excerpts from Fred Leeson, "Father's Tearful Pleas for His Child Eases His Wife's Sentence," *The Oregonian*, Saturday, April 17, 1993, Copyright © 1993, Oregonian Publishing Co. Used by permission of Oregonian Publishing Co.

Excerpts from Fred Leeson, "Reflections of a Shattered Relationship," *The Oregonian*, Saturday, August 7, 1993. Copyright © 1993. Oregonian Publishing Co. Used by permission of Oregonian Publishing Co.

Murray Straus, "Physical Assaults by Wives: A Major Social Problem," *Current Controversies on Family Violence*, edited by Richard J. Gelles and Donileen R. Loseke, pp. 67–87. Copyright © 1993 by Sage Publications, Inc. Reprinted by permission of Sage Publications, Inc., and Murray Straus; three graphic charts, used by permission of author.

Leslie J. Gregorash, "Family Violence: An Exploratory Study of Men Who Have Been Abused by Their Wives" (master's thesis, University of Calgary, 1993), p. 44. Used by permission of Leslie Gregorash.

Respecting Accuracy in Domestic Abuse Reporting, "Agenda for VAWA Reform." Published by RADAR, Washington, DC (2008), used by permission of authors.

Unpublished presentation of material presented at the National Family Violence Legislative Resource Center conference (February 2008, Sacramento, California) "From Ideology to Inclusion Evidence-Based Policy and Intervention in Domestic Violence." By Murray Straus, Ph.D. Courtesy of Murray A. Straus.

For Colin and Ethan.

May you inherit a more loving and peaceful world.

Contents

Tables and Figures

Acknowledgments

This book would not have been possible without the materials and many helpful suggestions of Murray Straus, Ph.D., and R. L. McNeely, Ph.D., J.D. Any mistakes in interpreting the research are mine, not theirs. This first chapter of this second edition was also particularly improved by graphic illustrations provided by Straus. The first edition of this volume would not have been completed without the assistance of John T. Harney of Book Consultants of Boston, and I am most grateful for his help. I luckily found Nancy Wolf, who provided essential professional help in preparing the final manuscript. Sue Steinmetz, Ph.D., and Coramae Mann, Ph.D., were particularly available for questions. Monique Hampton put time and energy into improving the first draft. Research assistant James Dixon's timely efforts were most helpful. My appreciation extends to Scot Thurman for preparing some of the graphic tables. Sharon Flues was helpful in a number of ways. Thanks as well to Gary Hankins, Ph.D., for his insights and stimulating influence. My thanks to Jim Cook (no relation) of the Joint Custody Association of California for his legislative research abstract of 1990, which initially helped to point me in the right direction for many of the sources cited here. This second edition was also particularly improved by the research and efforts of John Hamel, LCSW. I am also indebted to Cathy Young for use of portions of her article "Domestic Violence an In-Depth Analysis," originally posted on the Independent Women's Forum Web site, for some of the language and research sources in Chapter 5.

Introduction

This book is a first. There have been a number of published research articles regarding men who have been physically abused by their domestic partners and a few books with chapters on the subject, but no previous book had focused on this issue in a comprehensive way. Since the original publication in late 1997, several new books have been published, but this apparently remains the most comprehensive examination of the particular subject of abused men. It is noteworthy, however, that several books intended for an audience broader than an academic or professional one have emerged dealing with the issue of intimate personal violence from a holistic perspective. Even those who do not have a personal interest in male spousal abuse probably know someone who does. Beyond the main issue, I have also examined official and media reaction and have viewed the tactics to silence academic inquiry, as well as the social assumptions about the common behaviors of men and women. I have attempted to examine a wide range of public policy and to gather scattered research into one place. The cumulative results of this scientific study will likely astonish many readers. Social workers, attorneys, therapists, sociologists, criminologists, and other professionals are heard from in this book. It will provide assistance for helping professionals in their efforts to deal with a problem that must become more widely recognized.

It is important for the victims to know that they are not alone. I hope to help them by sharing the stories of real people from diverse sections of society. As predicted in the first edition, this book has generated controversy, but it has also sparked change. My hope remains that it will contribute to a rational discussion of a generally ignored area of domestic violence. Simply put, domestic violence in any form, by either gender, is wrong. How victims, perpetrators, helping professionals, and society in general deal with any such violence is the real issue. If we ignore one kind of violence and implicitly maintain that it should be ignored, other kinds of violence become more acceptable.

Looking at only one side of the domestic abuse equation is not the way to create appropriate public policy, and it does not reflect reality. I have attempted to contribute a new perspective on one facet of this multidimensional issue and to suggest some solutions.

Why did I choose this subject? For two decades of my professional life, I have been a daily news reporter, working mainly in large cities. I have also reported from smaller cities and towns, where every shooting murder and many police calls responding to violence meant that the news media was there, too, even if it did not always warrant a filed story. I have seen the body bags, the bullet holes, the blood, the broken bones, and the bruises. I have witnessed the arguments and cursing. I have seen the tearful, frightened children. Although I have not been a victim of domestic violence myself, nor was violence present in my family, I have seen enough of it to care deeply.

In the past, I came into contact with a number of victims of domestic violence—male and female—working with a charitable organization concerned with the effects of parental separation on children. Most of this group's work involved educational classes for separated parents, professional seminars, supervised visitation, support groups, and mediation. The organization often saw couples who were separating for mediation sessions. In most office visits, though, individual men and women are seen for legal consumer information and referrals. A standard question on the intake form was whether the client has been a victim of a physical attack by a domestic partner. I was astonished by the number of men who checked "yes" and their descriptions of the extent of the abuse. (For this book, I conducted more extensive follow-up interviews with these clients and other male victims around the country. I also gathered information on cases in Great Britain, Canada, and Australia.) I was surprised at how willing these men were to discuss with me—and female staff—what happened to them. A number of them were eager to talk about it because we were the first ever to ask. Because these men felt safe from ridicule, they unburdened themselves, often with an obvious feeling of relief. It was also clear that most of these victims had kept their history hidden from friends, coworkers, and new female partners. These victims need understanding and respect, which will not come about without recognition.

In a sense, this book is an examination of the hidden. It is a study of neglected research, a study of hidden abusers and their victims. It seeks to shed light on the group of helping professionals and social scientists who are proposing new ways of thinking about and dealing with domestic violence. It is a subject that should no longer remain hidden from men or women.

Chapter 1

Is It Real? The Evidence for a Significant Social Problem

There is no question that domestic violence directed against women is a serious problem. Former U.S. Surgeon General Dr. C. Everett Koop has called it women's number-one health problem. The statistics reported in the popular press are staggering; though they are not always reported accurately. The most frequently cited statistic is that a woman is beaten every 15 seconds by her intimate partner.

In light of these statistics, it may be difficult for most of us to accept that women assault men at anywhere near the rate that men assault women. If it happened frequently, wouldn't we hear more about it? Maybe it only occurs when an older, physically frail man is abused by a younger woman or when a woman has been assaulted or abused and is fighting back? Can injuries to men be very serious, since women are not generally as physically strong as men? These are a few of the most common questions surrounding this issue. We will take a look at these and other questions and discuss research findings.

This book can be utilized by a general readership, and at times, it directly challenges common assumptions about how men and women behave. It has implications for a broad spectrum of public policy as well as for the helping professions. Simple presentation of the data is not sufficient. It is necessary to go into detail about how the data were gathered, how they compare to other research, and the conclusions of these respected researchers.

For the purposes of this book, here are some definitions:

Violence: An act carried out with the intention, or perceived intention, of causing physical injury or pain to another person.

Minor violent acts: To throw something at another; to push, grab, shove, slap, or spank.

Severe violent acts: To kick, bite, or hit with a fist; to hit or try to hit with an object; to beat up the other; to threaten with a knife, gun, or other deadly weapon; to use a knife, gun, or other deadly weapon.

Abuse: Physical abuse or threat of physical abuse; using violence or carrying out violent acts.[1]

In this book, abuse is addressed in terms of physical abuse or the threat of physical violence. Psychological and sexual abuse are not generally addressed; although sexual abuse is discussed throughout, it is not the main focus. A forthcoming book will delve more deeply into this particular subject. For the most part, I have also chosen not to investigate gay man versus gay man violence (except in a limited comparison to lesbian versus lesbian violence), nonintimate relationship violence, elder abuse, or child abuse. Maintenance of a consistent focus necessitates imposing some conditions on the areas investigated.

Do women physically assault their mates on a scale similar to men? The answer often depends on who is asking the question, how it is asked, and how the data are analyzed. Statistical results from surveys can vary greatly owing to differences between the populations studied, so it is often best to directly examine results obtained from different reporting groups first in order to piece together an overall picture. It then becomes easier to judge these results fairly as they compare to more generally representative surveys.

WHAT THE SURVEYS SHOW

Police Reports

Incidents actually reported to police are certainly a starting point for examining the level of domestic violence in the United States and in other countries. Maureen McLeod appears to have conducted the most exhaustive examination of police records on spousal abuse. She reported her results in *Justice Quarterly*.[2] At the time of the study (1984), she was an assistant professor of criminal justice and the coordinator of the Women's Studies Program at Stockton State College in Pomona, New Jersey. McLeod examined over 6,000 spousal assault cases reported to the Detroit Police Department. She found that male reports of spousal assault made up 6 percent of the total number reported. This survey result is consistent with data gathered from two other localities that showed rates of police-reported male spousal assaults of 6 percent and 10 percent.[3] As we shall discuss a bit later in this chapter, the actual numbers of males now reporting spousal abuse to police have increased since the 1990s.

Although it does not measure actual police arrest rates, the National Crime Victimization Survey (NCVS) is labeled a crime survey and is conducted by the

U.S. Department of Justice (DOJ). In its survey for 1992–1993, which was redesigned to produce more accurate reporting of intimate crime than surveys of previous years, one million women and 143,000 men were victims of intimate violence. In previous studies, women reported an annual average of 572,032 spousal abuse cases, whereas men reported an annual average of 48,983 cases. Between 2001 and 2005, the average annual number of intimate crime cases declined again—dramatically for women, but less so for men: 511,000 women and 105,000 men, respectively. The total number of victimized women in this survey continues to show evidence of decline. Although there has also been somewhat of a decline in the number of victimized men, the relative percentage of male victims continues to increase over the years, for example, from 15 percent in 1993 to 17 percent in 2005. In addition:

- About 96 percent of females reporting nonfatal intimate partner violence were victimized by a male, and about 3 percent were victimized by another female.
- About 82 percent of males reporting nonfatal intimate partner violence were victimized by a female, and about 16 percent were victimized by another male.[4]

These numbers are far less than those most often reported in the news media. The NCVS also finds that police are more likely to make a formal report if the offender is a stranger than if the offender is an intimate. However, the survey still carries the burden of calling itself a *crime* survey and does not limit itself to asking solely questions about intimate violence. Unfortunately, after answering questions about such easily defined crimes as robbery, some victims may not categorize domestic violence as a crime. For this and other reasons, the DOJ survey may still fail to adequately represent the totality of domestic violence in the United States. Traditionally, a victim is more likely to report serious injury assaults by a former partner than to report assaults or injuries from a current live-in partner.[5] Also, the NCVS reports far fewer injuries by partners than another survey conducted by the DOJ, which reviews injuries reported in hospital emergency rooms.

Advocates at women's shelters have long maintained that there is consistent nonreporting by abused women to police and other authorities. McLeod found this is also true for abused men; in fact, she found that abused men fail to file police reports at an even greater rate than their female counterparts: "Whereas 54 percent of abused females claim they have notified the police of the assaultive incident, only 45 percent of the male victims allege they have taken this action."[6] McLeod also found that male victims are "significantly less likely than females to pursue prosecution once the police have been notified and the immediate need for intervention has subsided."[7] In a report published by the Police Foundation, six other researchers agreed with McLeod's findings in this regard.[8]

These results are consistent with DOJ figures reporting that males are 11 percent less likely than women to report *any* type of violent crime in which they were the victims.[9] Thus, police reports and crime victimization surveys alone do not give a complete picture of the incidence of domestic violence in the United States for women, and they are even less likely to do so for men. They are instructive mainly in giving us a picture of this reporting population.

Unfortunately, there is no comprehensive national survey of actual police arrests for domestic violence in the United States that lists the arrests by gender. Different police departments have different reporting methods, and apparently, the majority does not keep records of who was arrested by gender. However, I did find state and city totals for these types of arrests.

The results I report here must be qualified with this in mind: they are best estimates and should not be considered scientific nor the results of a comprehensive survey; they are averages of 15 small-to-large cities, plus one state-wide total:

> Domestic violence arrests of females averaged 20 percent of the total number of such arrests in the United States. The range, however, was wide. In Portland, Oregon, for example, the police department reported that female arrests were 14 percent of total arrests, while in the smaller city of Petaluma, California, the arrest rate for females was 23 percent.
>
> More than 10 years ago when research for this book was first conducted, the average arrest rate for women was about 6 percent, according to the few published research results available at the time.
>
> There seems to be no question that there has been a dramatic increase in female arrests in the past 10 years.

Why this is occurring will be discussed in Chapter 4.

Hospital Surveys

The problem with extrapolating results from a narrowly selected population group and applying them to the general public holds particularly true for the most widely reported study involving hospital emergency room admissions. The results were published in the *Journal of the American Medical Association in* 1984. Wendy Goldberg and Michael Tomlanovich surveyed patients seeking treatment at the Henry Ford Hospital emergency room in Detroit, Michigan, using a confidential, self-administered questionnaire. Twenty-two percent of the patients identified themselves as being victims of domestic violence. "More than half the subjects were hit or pushed, one-third had objects thrown at them or were kicked or threatened with harm, and approximately one-tenth were stabbed, whipped, or threatened with being killed."[10] The researchers noted: "The study did not find a statistically significant difference between the number of male and female domestic violence victims."[11] The relevant gender difference in this study related to perception and seeking help. Women viewed the relationship more negatively and requested counseling services more often. This study should be viewed with some caution in two regards. First, the questionnaire asked if "at some time" the person had been a victim of specific acts of domestic violence. So the abuse inquiry was not directly related to that specific hospital emergency room visit. Second, the research site was one Detroit hospital; hence, the results did not accurately represent hospitals nationwide.

One of the main reasons I wanted to update this book was because at the time of its original publication, there was no available comprehensive, nationally representative study of emergency room (ER) visits related to intimate partner violence that asked questions of both men and women. Now there is one, but only one. The total number of injuries reported in this ER survey is four times higher than that found in the NCVS, even though the DOJ conducts both surveys. This leads credence to the theory that the NCVS may underestimate the totality of the crime.

The ER survey results found that 60 percent of those injured for assaults of all types were male. Of all assaults, 17 percent were due to intimate partner violence. Of these, 14 percent were female victims, and 3 percent were male victims. The relationship to the assailant was unknown for one-fifth of the female victims and one-third of the male victims. Thus, even in this 70-hospital survey, where ER personnel were instructed to note and chart the assault victim's relationship, there was significant underreporting for females and highly significant underreporting for males. It should also be noted that one-third of men are less likely than women to seek treatment for injuries from any cause. In total, this report found that 243,000 people a year seek treatment in emergency rooms for injuries due to intimate partner violence, or 142, 094 women and 10,006 men.[12]

The ER survey did not find that intimate partner violence is the leading cause of injuries in emergency rooms, nor did it represent the majority of all assaults.

In Chapter 4 we will examine the many highly publicized and sometimes even official government pronouncements that domestic violence is the leading cause of injury to women.

Military Survey

An assumption involving another particular group and spousal abuse has become accepted, owing to the work of an early advocate for battered women. *Battered Wives* author Del Martin finds a direct correlation between military service and the likelihood of increased wife battering, although she admits that there is no empirical evidence: "The military is a school for violence....He is taught to idealize aggression and rugged masculinity....Is it far-fetched to think that there is a connection between military training or combat experience and wife-beating? I don't think so."[13] Martin's belief has been repeated elsewhere as an assumption that since the military is, by its nature, a regimented, hierarchical macho machine—although it is changing with more women in service—military men must be more dangerous to their wives. Until now, there have been no hard data one way or the other.

Using a Freedom of Information Act request, I obtained a copy of a huge survey of U.S. Army personnel regarding domestic violence, involving 55,000 randomly selected soldiers from 47 military installations. Male soldiers reported a rate of minor to severe violence of 29 to 34 percent. Female soldiers reported a rate of 39 to 40 percent. This rate is just as appalling as results from surveys of the general population, but the figures do not demonstrate a significantly higher level of domestic violence in the military as compared to society in general. The military report concludes: "The most common pattern is for physical aggression to be reported for both partners."[14] The military survey of those reporting violence in their relationship is divided into regional areas; however, Table 1.1 combines this data for clarity and ease of comparison.

There was a remarkable difference in the rate of violence between military installations. In the first regional area, consisting of 18 bases, the lowest rate of domestic violence was about 18 percent, while the highest rate was 48 percent. Exactly which bases these were remains a military secret, but the data strongly suggest that high-stress duty has more to do with domestic violence than the fact of military service per se. The author of the report supports this conclusion:

> There is a clear trend for personnel in the high [domestic violence] installations to report higher levels of stress symptoms, more unfavorable working conditions and in general, more marital disagreement. Additionally, there may be a relationship between the risk for marital violence and down-sizing, as the highest prevalence installation, which would in most other respects not be considered to be at high risk, is scheduled to be closed.[15]

Table 1.1
Perpetrator of Violence

	Spouse Only	Both Violent	Self Only	Total
Male soldiers	23%	62–64%	13–14%	8,500
Female soldiers	17–23%	60–64%	23%	1,246

Shelter Surveys

Many reports have been published regarding domestic violence based on interviews with a select population—women who have gone to shelters or called hotlines. R. L. McNeely and Gloria Robinson-Simpson, reporting in *Social Work,* contend that these surveys are of doubtful value in obtaining a picture of the overall level of domestic violence:

> Data collected and conclusions drawn from those who seek shelter or therapy cannot be generalized to the broader population. Victims who seek services may differ significantly from the broader population, so the value of these studies lies primarily in spawning clinical prescriptions for treatment, not in describing or explaining domestic violence in general.[16]

It is instructive to note that in the few cases where residents of women's shelters were asked if they had been violent toward their mates, women did admit to a significant level of violence. Jean Giles-Sims's *Wife Battering: A Systems Theory Approach* reports that in the year before coming to the shelter, 77 percent of the women said they had been violent toward their partners. This number decreased to 42 percent within six months after leaving the shelter. Fifty-eight percent of the women's shelter residents reported that they had been violently abusive), whereas only 17 percent reported abusive violence against their partners after leaving the shelter. While some of these assaults could have been in self-defense (the survey did not ask this question directly), it is doubtful that all of them were. Giles-Sims reports:

> Some of the women also had been violent in the year before they came to the shelter. Over half had acted in ways that could cause serious injury to the man. Unfortunately, we cannot compare the extent of injury to each of the people involved in these relationships because the men were not interviewed.[17]

A survey sponsored by the Law Enforcement Assistance Administration of abused women seeking shelter in Kentucky found that among violent couples, 38 percent of the attacks were by women against men. The women said they initiated that percentage of the violence.[18]

A 1975 survey of the world's first shelter for abused women, located in England, found that of the 400 women questioned, 82.5 percent participated in a mutually violent relationship. A different survey of 100 women at this same shelter found that 62 percent were violence prone and that they were both the victims and the perpetrators of regular acts of violence. Some were more violent than the men they were seeking shelter from, according to the shelter's founder, Erin Pizzey.[19]

These shelter results, while limited, do act as a signpost toward accepting the reports of violent women in more comprehensive surveys.

General Population and National Surveys

The results of the first comprehensive survey of violent family life, based on a general nationally representative sample, was originally made available to the public in 1977, then published in book form in 1980. *Behind Closed Doors: Violence in the American Family* was written by Murray Straus, Richard Gelles, and Suzanne Steinmetz. At the time the book was written, Straus was a professor of sociology at the University of New Hampshire, Gelles taught sociology at the University of Rhode Island and was chair of the department, and Steinmetz was at the University of Delaware College of Home Economics. Another early study was conducted by Linda Nisonoff, a clinical psychologist at State University of New York at Stony Brook, and Irving Bitman, a sociologist at Fordham University. They published "Spouse Abuse: Incidence and Relationship to Selected Demographic Variables," which appeared in *Victimology* in 1979.

The first book about battered wives was published in 1974. Erin Pizzey's *Scream Quietly or the Neighbors Will Hear* is generally credited with starting the modem women's movement against domestic violence. Another early, influential book was Del Martin's *Battered Wives*, first published in 1976 and updated in 1983.

It is apparent by the dates of their original work that Straus, Gelles, and Steinmetz were very early in examining the issue of domestic violence. It is also notable that Martin, among other feminist writers, has referred to their research frequently. In fact, Martin refers to these three as "sociologists who have contributed greatly to our knowledge of wife-beating as a social phenomenon in the United States."[20]

Indeed, the most widely reported figures on domestic violence—4 million women a year in the United States suffering domestic violence by their partners and 1.8 million women seriously assaulted—comes from the Straus/ Gelles surveys. These same sources report an equal number of men experiencing domestic violence and an even greater number (two million) being seriously assaulted. These surveys were conducted at the University of New Hampshire and supported by funding from the National Institute of Mental Health (NIMH). The most widely accepted figures of two million women severely assaulted are quite often reported in the popular media as resulting in one woman being battered by her spouse every 15 seconds. The source is often erroneously cited as the Federal Bureau of Investigation or the DOJ, who consistently report figures much less than that amount. More precise and balanced results from the most recent National Family Violence Survey reveal *a woman being severely assaulted every 17.5 seconds and man being severely assaulted every 15.7 seconds.* The data on male spousal abuse are generally not cited. Chapter 4 will examine this "selective inattention"[21] in detail.

When this book was first published, there were at least 30 scientific studies supporting the results of Straus, Gelles, and Steinmetz. As of this writing, there are over 200 published peer-reviewed studies coming to the same essential conclusion: that women and men in intimate relationships assault each other at equal rates and initiate assaults at equal rates. Figure 1.1 gives a good picture of these published studies. There is one exception to this result. One major national survey did not find roughly equal rates but found that 36 percent of victims were male. We will discuss this result in detail just a bit later in this chapter.

It is instructive first to consider the early survey by Nisonoff and Bitman. They used a simple telephone poll that resulted in 297 completed questionnaires:

> 25 percent of the men and 16.5 percent of the women reported having hit or been hit by their mate. Fifty percent of those who had been hit had also hit their spouse....To assess whether housewives were more likely candidates for abuse, married female respondents were divided into "working

Figure 1.1
Cumulative Number of Studies Showing Similar Rates of Assaulting a Partner by Women and Men

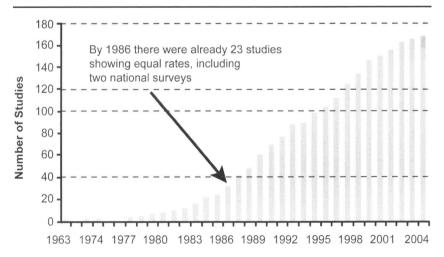

Note: From Murray Straus, Ph.D., Co-Director Family Research Laboratory, University of New Hampshire, presentation to the National Family Violence Legislative Center conference "From Ideology to Inclusion," Sacramento, California, February, 2008. Courtesy of Murray A. Straus.

wives" and "homemakers"; 13.1 percent of the former and 11.3 percent of the latter reported being hit by their spouse....There was no trend for less-educated women to report more frequently being abused. Alcohol was a contributing factor in 26 percent of the violent incidents...[N]o sex differences were found in frequency or severity....Wives reported hitting their husbands almost as frequently as husbands reported hitting wives, and a higher proportion of men reported having been hit by their wives than vice versa....[The] theory that coercive behavior tends to be reciprocated between spouses is supported by our finding that 50 percent of the couples reporting spousal violence had both hit and been hit by their mate....Divorced and separated persons, as expected, were much more likely to report having been hit, and somewhat more likely to...[report having] hit their spouse, than were other respondents.[22]

The scope of the Straus/Gelles work makes the 297 people surveyed by Nisonoff/Bitman appear sparse. The results, however, are comparable. The NFVS, supported with funding by the NIMH, looked at nationally representative samples of 2,143 married and cohabiting couples in 1975 and 6,002 couples in 1985.[23]

We can see from the data shown in Table 1.2 that the rates of overall spousal violence are nearly equal. The good news is that the rate of violence against women by men decreased in the 10 years between surveys; the bad news is that the rate of violence against men stayed nearly the same or increased.

Owing to severe criticism by some, Straus reexamined the data in 1993 in order to remove any possibility of gender bias in reporting. He compared the rates in the general survey to the reports given solely by women. In other words, what did the women say about their own assaults against their mates? He found no difference: "As these rates are based exclusively on information provided by women respondents, the near equality in assault rates cannot be attributed to a gender bias in reporting."[24]

The comprehensive surveys in the United States have been replicated elsewhere, most notably in Canada. In a report published in a German sociological

Table 1.2
Rate of Violence per 1,000 Couples

	1975	1985
Husband against wife		
Overall violence	121	113
Severe violence	38	30
Wife against husband		
Overall violence	116	121
Severe violence	46	44

journal, Eugen Lupri conducted a national survey from the University of Calgary in which 1,123 usable questionnaires were returned. The 652 females and 471 males participating were those who were currently or previously married or cohabiting. The Canadian researchers utilized a slightly modified Conflict Tactics Scale, used by Straus/Gelles, which Lupri called valid, widely used, and reliable.[25] The results were similar to those in the United States:

> Approximately 2.5% of men and 6.2% of women admitted to having beaten up their partners. In the overall violence index, and in the severe violence index, women reported more acts: 18% of the men and 23% of the women reported overall violence against their mate, while 10% of the men and 13% of the women reported severe violence. The rates for actually using a knife or gun against a mate were nearly identical, 0.5% for men, 0.7% for women. On the basis of approximately 5.9 million couples in Canada in 1986, the Overall Violence Index of 17.8 for men and 23.3 for women means that conservatively speaking, over 1 million husbands and wives engaged in some form of physical violence....An important finding of our national study is that legally married or cohabitating women and men who abuse their intimate partners come from all regions of the country, communities, age groups, educational backgrounds, income levels, and occupations.[26]

Lupri and a number of other researchers contend that women are more likely to self-report their own acts of violence, while men are more likely to underreport their acts because men are more culturally accepting of violence and are more likely to deny or minimize the seriousness of the abuse. Lupri says women do this, too: "In an attempt to keep the peace and to reduce the likelihood of further harm, a woman also minimizes and denies the seriousness of the abuse and frequently does not challenge the man's inadequate explanations."[27]

Whether this is true when women fill out a confidential, self-administered questionnaire is open to question. It is also questionable whether men tend more often than women do to underreport such violent acts in surveys. Certainly, the way the questions were framed in the Canadian survey (Figure 1.2) would give both men and women as much freedom as possible to answer them honestly:

> No matter how well spouses or partners get along, there are times when they disagree on major decisions, are annoyed with what the other person does, or are simply in a bad mood or tired. At the left is a list of things you might have done when you had a conflict or disagreement with your partner. Please circle a number for each of the things in the list, showing how often you did it in the past year or in the last year of your marriage.[28]

This statement seems to be saying that everybody does it, even if only because a person is in a bad mood. Given the great deal of public attention and press

Figure 1.2
Canadian Survey Reports of Domestic Violence

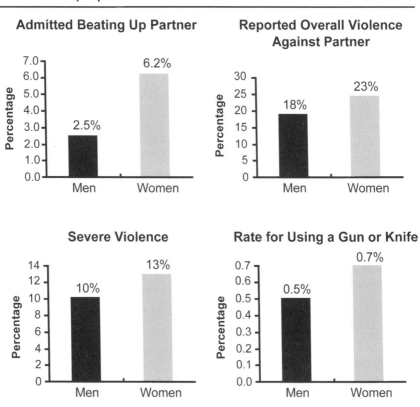

related to domestic violence against women, it does seem probable that men would be more likely to underreport their own acts, no matter how gently the questions are framed. Men also tend to minimize or downplay violent acts committed against them. Since there has been virtually no censure of women for violent domestic acts against their partners, however, it would not seem that women would underreport acts against their partners or their mate's violent actions against them. Statistics Canada also reports a similar rate of domestic violence in a much larger survey of more than 11,000 men and women, finding that 8 percent of women and 7 percent of men suffered from intimate partner abuse.

It is not particularly valuable to list in this book all of the domestic violence research, especially given the fact that there are over 200 surveys now published. However, the resources section at the end of this book provides a Web site, maintained by Martin Fiebert, Ph.D., at the University of California at Long Beach, which lists all the published results.

Most interesting, perhaps, in terms of new information, is comparison data about college-age students for some 30 countries (see Table 1.3, which includes results from the international dating survey). The results found equal or nearly equal rates of intimate partner assaults between young men and women (Table 1.4). The "macho" or male patriarchy theory as a cause of domestic violence is called into question, because there was no difference in the rates of Latin American countries compared with rates in the United States.

We come now to the National Violence Against Women Survey (NVAWS). When this book was first published, this report had not yet been conducted. This survey was funded by the DOJ and the Centers for Disease Control (CDC). It was conducted by the Center for Policy Research, and the lead author was Patricia Tjaden, Ph.D.[29]

Table 1.3
Ten Other Examples of the Approximately 200 Studies Showing Gender Symmetry in Assault

Study	Severity of Assault	Perpetrator	
		Male	**Female**
Canadian National Survey (Lupri, 1990)	Severe	17.8%	23.3%
	Minor	10.1%	12.9%
Canadian General Social Survey (1999)	Overall rate	7.0%	8.0%
British Crime Survey (1996)	Overall rate	4.2%	4.1%
National Comorbidity Study (Kessler, 2001)	Minor	17.4%	17.7%
	Severe	6.5%	6.2%
National Alcohol and Family Violence Survey (Straus, 1995)	Overall rate	9.1%	9.5%
	Severe	1.9%	4.5%
Dunedin Health and Development Study (US Dept of Justice, 1999)	Overall rate	27.0%	34.0%
National Violence Against Women Survey (Tjaden & Thoennes, 2000)	Overall rate	1.3%	0.9%
Youth Risk Behavior Survey (Centers For Disease Control, 2006)	Overall rate	8.8%	8.9%
National Youth Survey (Wofford-Mihalic, Elliott, & Menard, 1994)	Overall	20.2%	34.1%
	Severe	5.7%	3.8%
Percent of Emergency room visits for PV (Ernst et al., *Annals of Emergency Medicine,* 1997)		19.0%	20.0%

Note: From Murray Straus, Ph.D., Co-Director Family Research Laboratory, University of New Hampshire, presentation to the National Family Violence Legislative Center conference "From Ideology to Inclusion," Sacramento, California, February, 2008. Courtesy of Murray A. Straus.

Table 1.4
Five of the 17 General Population Studies Showing Mutual Violence Predominates

Study	Among Violent Couples		
	Both violent	Male only	Female only
1. National Family Violence Survey, 1975	48%	25%	27%
2. National Comorbidity Survey, 1990–2002	54%	23%	24%
3. National Long. Study of Adolescent Health, 2001	50%	15%	35%
4. International Dating Violence Study, 2001–2006	55%	16%	29%
5. International Parenting Study, 2008	60%	11%	29%

All 17 Studies Show that Mutual Violence Predominates

1. Straus, M. A., Gelles, R. J., & Steinmetz, S. K. (1980 [2006]). *Behind closed doors: Violence in the American family* New York: Doubleday/Anchor Books (Re-issued Transaction Publications, 2006 with a new foreword by Richard J. Gelles and Murray A. Straus).
2. As reported by women. Kessler, R. C., Molnar, B. E., Feurer, I. D., & Appelbaum, M. (2001). Patterns and mental health predictors of domestic violence in the United States: Results from the National Comorbidity Survey. *International Journal of Law And Psychiatry, 24*(4–5), 487–508.
3. Third wave, when age 19-23. Whitaker, D. J., Haileyesus, T., Swahn, M., & Saltzman, L. S. (2007). Intimate partner violence. *American Journal of Public Health, 97*(5), 941-947.
4. University students in 32 nations. Straus, M. A. (2007, in press). Dominance and symmetry in partner violence by male and female university students in 32 nations. *Children and Youth Services Review.*

Note: From Murray Straus, Ph.D., Co-Director Family Research Laboratory, University of New Hampshire, presentation to the National Family Violence Legislative Center conference "From Ideology to Inclusion," Sacramento, California, February, 2008. Courtesy of Murray A. Straus.

In an interview with the author, Dr. Tjaden said, "Well, this must be a good survey since neither side was happy."

What she meant was that while the survey gave a lower percentage of male victims than the University of New Hampshire National Violence Survey of about 10 years earlier (1985 vs. 1995-results published in 2000), it also *lowered* the total number of victimized women (from 1.8 million a year to 1.5 million a year). The total number of victimized men was given at 885,000 a year, or 36 percent of the total number of victims. The definitions of assault were very similar to those of the earlier surveys, and these results reflect the total number of *severe* attacks.

There is no doubt that this survey was large and comprehensive, interviewing 16,000 men and women in all states. It was, however, a telephone survey, rather than using the self-administered questionnaire format. There were also questions about sexual assault in intimate partner settings that the National Family Violence Survey (NFVS) did not conduct, as well as questions about stalking. The NVAWS found that women are injured about twice as often as are men according to these self-reports (41.5% vs. 19.9%).

It is not my purpose, nor would it be very interesting for the general reader, to go into the details of the current sociological debate about the validity of these findings compared to the NFVS or other surveys. Suffice it to say that there is debate over telephone methods versus questionnaires and whether adding stalking questions influenced partner violence questions, and whether asking questions related to sexual abuse skewed the results. I will, however, examine the findings a bit more closely in regard to lesbian versus lesbian violence for a particular reason that will be explained later in the book.

I do not necessarily disagree with Tjaden's statement that since neither side was happy, it must be a good survey.

The data from the Violence Against Women Survey is interesting and valuable and is—curiously—fairly consistent (though a considerably higher percentage) with the average number of actual arrests of women.

As the title of the survey suggests (The National Violence Against *Women* Survey), it certainly cannot be construed to be a survey designed to be favorable to reports of male victimization. It does stand in contrast, however, to the majority of published reports on intimate partner violence that have consistently found an equal number of male and female victims.

The report did spark some media interest (e.g., CNN interviewed the author), with the majority of the news media describing it as a CDC report and mentioning the fact that it found a yearly average of 885,000 male victims of intimate partner violence in the United States.

Nearly as large as the NVAWS, and apparently at the time of this writing the most large scale (11,000 men and women), is a survey conducted primarily by Harvard researchers and published in the *American Journal of Public Health* in 2007:

> Almost 25% of the people surveyed—28% of women and 19% of men—said there was some violence in their relationship. Women admitted perpetrating more violence (25% versus 11%) as well as being victimized more by violence (19% versus 16%) than men did. According to both men and women, 50% of this violence was reciprocal, that is, involved both parties, and in those cases the woman was more likely to have been the first to strike.
>
> Violence was more frequent when both partners were involved, and so was injury—to either partner. In these relationships, men were more likely than women to inflict injury (29% versus 19%). When the violence was one-sided, both women and men said that women were the perpetrators about 70% of

the time. Men were more likely to be injured in reciprocally violent relationships (25%) than were women when the violence was one-sided (20%).[30]

That means both men and women agreed that men were not more responsible than women for intimate partner violence. The findings cannot be explained
by men's being ashamed to admit hitting women, because women agreed with
men on this point.

In summary, whether one accepts the NVAWS, NFVS, or *Journal of Public
Health* survey, or the hundreds of other survey results, the *least* that can be said
is that male victims represent 36 percent of the total number of domestic violence victims in the United States.

It must be noted, however, that there is a provable and consistent pattern
in the majority of domestic violence awareness or service organizations and
many official government agencies of considerable "cherry picking" in reporting these various results to achieve a desired end: overestimate the number
of abused women and downplay or ignore the number of abused men and
sometimes, though much more rarely, the reverse. We will explore more on
this issue in Chapter 4.

The data in the NVAWS or other surveys can and should be debated by those
with expertise in the area; however, it is the supporting language in the actual
NVAWS report by Tjaden and her coauthor that I find most disturbing, not so
much for what it said, but what it did not say.

Throughout the authors emphasize that the primary emphasis for prevention, treatment, and prosecution should be on intimate partner violence
against women due to the greater incidence of injury. There is nothing wrong
with that statement, and indeed, many others and I agree wholeheartedly with
it. We can debate whether or not in the most severe of the severe incidents men
are as likely to be injured when weapons, scalding liquids, and thrown hard
objects are used; in those cases, the evidence does seem to suggest a nearly
equal rate of injury. In McLeod's police report study, for example, 63 percent
of the men faced a deadly weapon, while only 15 percent of the women did. We
can also debate whether or not the survey should have added questions likely
to elicit more response from men, such as classifying being kicked or hit in the
groin as a sexual assault.

Primary emphasis, however, is quite different from exclusive emphasis. Not
one time, in the published report did Tjaden mention, reference, or even allude
to this statement, which I elicited from her in an interview: "The primary
emphasis should be placed on women due to the greater number of injuries.
Certainly, however, the results show a significant number of male victims and
the results should not be taken to mean that there should not be concern and
resources for them." I'll leave it up to those readers willing to read the entire

published report or even its shorter summary to see whether or not the same conclusion I came to is reached: the supporting language contains no statement of support or even any mention of the fact that concern and resources are lacking for men or are needed—despite what the data shows.

Having this picture of domestic violence from the various particular and general surveys now permits a more informed examination of certain assumptions that have led to the figures on male spousal abuse being disregarded, ignored, or downplayed.

MUTUAL ABUSE AND CONTEXT

The most often cited reason for ignoring the higher or nearly equal rate of domestic violence against men is that the figures include women acting in self-defense. This is not true in the majority of cases. Mutual combat is the norm in violent households. About 50 percent of those surveyed report both spouses to be violent. The remainder is nearly equally divided. In somewhat over a quarter of the cases (27 percent), the male was violent. About one-fourth of the time (24 percent), the female was violent, according to the Straus/Gelles surveys. (See Figure 1.3 for mutual combat results from a variety of studies.)

Figure 1.3
Mutual Combat

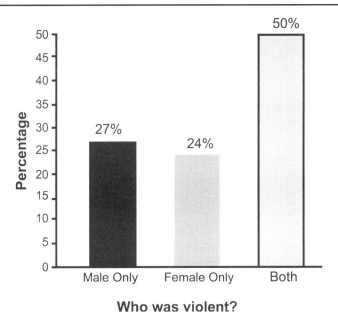

The *Journal of Public Health* authors also found similar results about mutually combative couples in their large nationwide survey.

Even if the results are focused only on "severe violence," the results come out about the same: both, 35 percent; husband only, 35.2 percent; and wife only, 29.6 percent.[31]

Mutual Combat

Straus comments:

> Regardless of whether the analysis is based on all assaults or is focused on dangerous assaults, about as many women as men attacked spouses who had not hit them, during the one-year referent period. This is inconsistent with the self-defense explanation for the high rate of domestic assault by women.
>
> However, it is possible that, among the couples where both assaulted, all the women were acting in self-defense. Even if that unlikely assumption were correct, it would still be true that 25–30% of violent marriages are violent solely because of attacks by the wife.[32]

The "unlikely assumption" about mutually violent couples was tested by the researchers at the Family Research Laboratory. They asked a large sample of wives in this category about who hit first. The women said they hit first 53 percent of the time, while their partners hit first 42 percent of the time. Three percent said they could not remember who hit first.

In examining these NFVS results, McNeely and Robinson-Simpson conclude that self-defense is not an adequate explanation for the high levels of violence reported for women: "Although the data do not indicate what proportion of the violent acts were in response to violent acts by men, the fact that women had higher mean and median rates for severe violence suggests that female aggression is not merely a response to male aggression."[33]

These results were reported in the first edition of this book. However, those who are intent on downplaying or ignoring the subject of abused men tend to say that there are no results such as these being reported or that the data revealed fails to put things "in context." I've heard the "in context" argument many times at various domestic violence conferences I have attended since this book's first edition. For example, Katherine Van Wormer from the University of Northern Iowa has published numerous domestic violence articles, and she wrote a review of the first edition on Amazon.com, saying, "Also on the battering statistics these figures include a lot of women slapping men who get fresh with them. Or self-defense assaults. So the facts revealed in this book and carried by the media are false."[34]

I'll leave the reader to their own conclusions as to whether a woman should always be given the liberty to slap a man for "getting fresh." For myself, I tend to be an absolutist about violence and don't think it's acceptable. Besides, a woman who slaps a man for any reason except self- defense only increases her chances of getting hit in return...it ultimately doesn't make her feel very good either. Be that as it may, had Van Wormer and other apologists for violent women actually taken the time to look at the data in this book's first edition (apparently Van Wormer did not) and from many other sources, they would find that self-defense as an explanation for domestic violence has been studied by a number of researchers. Indeed, it is this aspect of such situations that gives us the clearest picture of whole truth about domestic violence. The research also squares with the anecdotal experience of veteran police officers. Half of domestic violence involves mutual combat. People involved can't even remember very well who started it, but when they do (even when accepting only the woman's viewpoint), there is agreement; a quarter of the time only the woman was violent, a quarter of the time only the man was violent, women struck the first blow or threw something nearly half the time, the other half of the time the man did.

Personal accounts from those with a violent family life support this assertion. James, a 40-year-old man, describes his mother's attacks against his father and their mutual battles:

"She would, 99 times out of 100, throw the first punch, throw the first object. They got into some knock-down, drag-out battles, some actual physical hitting of each other. I remember my mother one time went into the kitchen and got a thing of vinegar out of the cabinet, poured a glass, and walked back to my father and threw a glass of vinegar in his face."[35]

In this case, while James describes attacks primarily initiated by his mother, it is notable that the battles usually ended up with both partners physically hitting each other. It might be assumed that even in the predominate case of mutual abuse among violent couples, any injuries that resulted would be more serious for the woman, given the male's generally greater physical strength. This assumption is challenged by some researchers and supported by others.

INJURIES

In her study of police records, McLeod found that 72 percent of the attacks against women by men involved the use of bodily force (hitting, punching, slapping, kicking, etc.), but for women assaulting men, only 14 percent involved bodily force, and only 15 percent of the women faced a gun or a knife in a domestic battle. A gun or a knife was used or threatened against a male victim 63 percent of the time. McLeod commented on this result from her survey and what others have reported:

The increased use of deadly weapons, and of knives in particular, by female assailants has been documented by other researchers. Wolfgang, in his study of homicides in Philadelphia, observed that knives and cutting objects were used four times as often by women as by men....One examination of reports of aggravated assaults in 17 cities [noted that]: "although there were fewer female assaulters than males, women would appear more dangerous than men when they actually become offenders."[36]

Alan, a 31-year-old Canadian man, offers some dramatic evidence of this type of assault:

> She'd do things like if she'd get mad enough, like she'll kick me right from behind, you know, right in the scrotum from behind. Just wam—unexpectedly. Or, you know, a couple of times she's used scissors. You know, you have to defend yourself against bloody hair cutting scissors, you know?[37]

Owing to greater use of cutting objects and other weapons, McLeod states, "Offenses against men are significantly more serious in nature than are offenses against women."[38] Her examination of police reports found, "Whereas just over one-fourth of all spouse abuse incidents involving female victims are categorized as aggravated assaults, the corresponding statistic for male victims is demonstrably higher...86% are aggravated; over two-thirds of these aggravated events are serious assaults with a weapon."[39] McLeod says the evidence shows

Figure 1.4
Use of Bodily Force

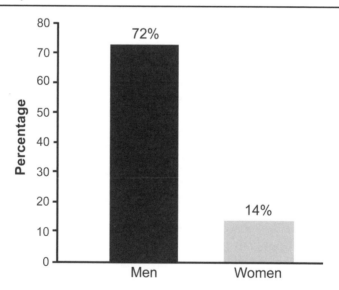

Note: Adapted from M. McLeod, "Women against Men: An Examination of Domestic Violence Based on an Analysis of Official Data and National Victimization Data," *Justice Quarterly* 1, 1984: 185.

that women are much more likely to have serious injury from kicking and hitting rather than from having a weapon used, while men are not very likely at all to have a serious injury from a hitting or kicking type of an assault.[40]

The more frequent use of weapons by women (82% for women vs. 25% for men) in spousal assaults results in a greater injury rate for men (Figures 1.4 and 1.5), according to McLeod: 77 percent of the assaulted men report some injury. "These statistics clearly exceed estimates of the extent of victim injury among female victims, generally documented as between 52 and 57 percent."[41] In fact, McLeod says, 84 percent of the men who were injured by domestic violence required medical attention, with 50 percent of these being hospitalized overnight or longer.

Straus, in reviewing this report, says that while the facts are fine, he does not agree with the interpretation that women engaged in more dangerous attacks and therefore inflicted more serious injury. Straus says, "My interpretation is that this is an artifact of what gets reported. Attacks by women, like attacks by men, are overwhelmingly 'minor violence.' The main difference is that attacks

Figure 1.5
Facing a Deadly Weapon (Guns and Knives)

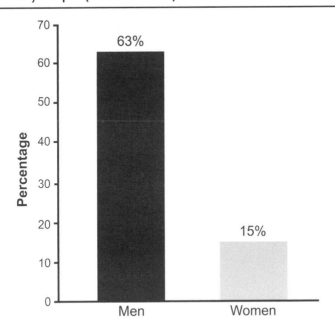

Note: Adapted from M. McLeod, "Women against Men: An Examination of Domestic Violence Based on an Analysis of Official Data and National Victimization Data," *Justice Quarterly* 1, 1984: 185.

by women tend to be reported only if they are truly dangerous and/or if an injury actually occurred."[42] He points out that an analysis of the NFVS found that attacks by men are about seven times more likely to result in an injury that requires medical treatment. The NVAWS found that women were about twice as likely to be injured. How can both arguments be right? By viewing them in a combined manner. That is, males may suffer serious injury more often, whereas females likely suffer a greater number of total injuries ranging from minor to serious. This is consistent with observations by Angela Browne of the University of Massachusetts Medical School that abused women tend to have several injuries to multiple sites of the body, while this kind of pattern is not seen in abused men. In other words, most domestic violence (by about a two-to-one margin) involves physical contact in which the male's greater physical strength comes into play—pushing, grabbing, shoving, slapping, spanking—while most female violence in this category involves throwing things. These types of physical acts of aggression toward a female by a male are more likely to result in injury requiring medical attention than the same type of physical acts by a female toward a male. The woman is unlikely to injure the man unless her aim is accurate, which is further impeded by the emotions of the moment.

The cautions previously observed regarding the victim-reporting reliability of police reports should mean some discounting of the overwhelmingly greater number of male injuries surveyed by McLeod. On the other hand, given the national survey results throughout the world that women engage in serious violence (where weapons as well as physical prowess come into play) to an equal or greater extent than men, we can suggest that the serious injury totals in this category are somewhat more equal for the genders.

A study by Barbara Morse at the Institute of Behavioral Science at the University of Colorado published in *Violence and Victims* found only a small difference between the total number of men and women who said they had sought medical attention for a domestic violence injury. A total of 13.5 percent of men and 20 percent of women said they suffered injury, and 14 percent of the men and 12 percent of the women said they sought medical care. More than one thousand people were surveyed. Women also said they initiated force 50 percent more often than men.[43] It may well be that abusive men are more likely than abusive women to engage in violence that results in multiple injuries due to repeated blows with a fist. The pattern for abusive women seems to be to throw something or to use a weapon but to strike with the fist less often within the incident. Thus, multiple injuries for men may be less common, but single injuries caused by objects and weapons and scalding liquids can still be serious enough to require medical attention and may be even be life-threatening more often than injuries caused by the heavy hand of the male. This study is of particular value because it asked more detailed questions about the type and result of the attack than did the larger ER study by the DOJ. It could well be true that most medical personnel simply do not know how to recognize male abuse. The fact that there was a much greater proportion of unavailable information about men compared to women in the ER study indicates that this is likely.

I am not aware of any comprehensive survey of medical personnel about comparative diagnosis procedures and views regarding male victims. The observational research, however, should be plain to everyone. In the doctor's office there are frequently brochures and small resource cards prominently available to someone with a domestic violence issue. The problem, of course, is that there are no brochures and most likely no local resources for abused men. Domestic violence awareness founder Erin Pizzey is among many who believe that medical personnel do not know what signs to look for and often do not think to ask their male patients about the source of injuries as being possibly inflicted by their mate. In particular, physicians may fail to ask questions about eye injuries (due to thrown glass or ceramic objects), burn injuries, "accidental" poisonings, and groin area injuries due to an attempted or successful kick or slug to the testicles.

Curiously, most surveys do not ask questions about a frequent form of attack reported by men, the use of scalding liquids or even poisons. I had an interesting phone conversation with a long-retired New York City police officer. In the early 1940s he was a rookie and responded with his partner to a "domestic disturbance." While climbing the stairs to the apartment, his partner saw a woman standing on a landing with a saucepan in her hands. To his astonishment, his partner pulled his gun and ordered the woman to carefully put the pan down. Contrary to common perception and TV shows, some officers can go their entire careers and only display their weapon a few times. So, this was extraordinary. Later, the veteran officer explained that another officer had been severely burned in the face when a woman threw a pan full of lye-laced oatmeal (lye was a common household ingredient for soap and washing clothes at the time) at the officer. Apparently, it was not uncommon for women wishing to kill or incapacitate their husbands to feed them the lye-laced oatmeal.

It may simply be a difference between the most common styles of attack for women and men, but the result comes out about the same: injury and intimidation.

Injury reports increase our recognition of all domestic violence as a serious social issue. It is important to remember that men as well as women are likely to have injuries due to domestic violence, especially when we consider that there are no "rules" in these battles. For example, R. L. McNeely recounts the story of a man who was rolled up in his bedsheets while asleep one night, then beaten repeatedly with a baseball bat.[44] More typical of these encounters is this description of general incidents by an abused man: "The argument would escalate into a fight and then she would get violent. She would grab anything that was around. I went through three phones in one year. She would take and throw it or anything that was around."[45] The majority of domestic violence surveys find that women are nearly twice as likely to throw things and significantly more likely to kick or hit with an object.[46]

The old stereotype of a husband getting a plate thrown at him or being hit over the head with a rolling pin or frying pan is all too true. While some people may think of such an image as humorous (see Chapter 4), this type of aggression often does result in serious injury.

Here are two representative human stories of such abuse. They are unusual in that not only have they been verified by the historical record, they are the only examples of domestic violence (others have been suspected but disproved by historians) in this particular location, and nearly everyone in the world knows something about the house they lived in and the two couples.

Abe was a very tall man, somewhat thin, but in fairly good shape still from his days as a young man splitting wood. Mary Todd, his wife, was short even for a woman at the time and somewhat plump. She would frequently belittle him even in front of others, denigrate his efforts, and also sometimes fly into uncontrollable rages, hitting him with her fists and kicking him. Sometimes she would throw as heavy a piece of firewood that she could find. If one of those pieces of firewood had hit at just the right spot, John Wilkes Booth would not be a famous name today.

Bill had a sexual liaison with an intern in his office. When he finally had to admit publicly that it was true, his wife, Hillary, slapped him hard enough to leave a red mark on the side of his head that was clearly visible to others. A lamp may also have been thrown.[47]

There have been some interesting reactions to this true story in an informal public opinion survey, which we shall explore further in Chapter 5.

In examining domestic violence overall and whether men represent a significant portion of those abused, the ultimate form of abuse cannot be ignored.

FEMALE MURDERERS

What about women who kill? Domestic homicides show yearly fluctuations. The DOJ studied the rates for 1979 through 1988 and found that about 20 percent more females than males were slain by their mates. The figures for 1988 perhaps are the most accurate, as the Bureau of Justice Statistics surveyed a larger-than-usual number of homicides, about 8,000 in 75 large urban areas. The results of this survey, not released until 1994, show that of all white family murder victims, 62 percent were wives and 38 percent were husbands. In African American families, "wives were just about as likely to kill their husbands as husbands were to kill their wives: 47% of the victims of a spouse were husbands and 53% were wives." For both black and white victims, about 40 percent of the men and 60 percent of the women were killed by their spouses. From another perspective, during 1988, 216 men were killed by their wives, whereas 311 women were killed by their husbands.[48]

Almost 10 years later, in 1996, 1,800 murders were attributed to intimates, which represented a sharp decline (36%) from nearly 3,000 in 1976. In 1996, three in every four victims of intimate murder were female. The sharpest decrease from prior years was in the number of black male victims.

The yearly fluctuations in murder rates and the effect of changing economic times, age of the population, and how the homicide rate is measured among other factors means that it is difficult to say with precision what the intimate partner murder rate actually is at any given time.

The numbers show that a woman is nearly 25 percent more likely than a man to be killed by her mate. Murder rates show yearly fluctuations, which is why it is important to examine DOJ reports that combine and average periods over five years. In the last 15 years, there has been a remarkable stability, which first came to light in the 1980s. In other words, the difference of about 20–25 percent (except among black couples) has remained fairly constant. What is important to note, however, is that prior to this period, there was no difference. Wives killed husbands at about the same rate as husbands killed wives. Why the change? According to Katherine Van Wormer from the University of Northern Iowa, in a review of this book on Amazon.com: "What people need to realize is that women's shelters are saving the lives of more men than women. Read my analysis of the government statistics from the [United States] and Canada to see why this is so. (See Counseling Female Offenders and Victims, 2001). Women are not murdering men like they were due to the fact that they were killing out of fear. Now they have the shelter option."[49] First, the reason women murder their husbands is not always due to fear. (This is explored in detail in the first edition of my book.) In fact, a comprehensive examination by Coramae Mann and detailed below found that the majority of female spouse killers do not murder out of fear or self-defense. Some murder out of greed, others because they've taken a new lover and find murder a way to get rid of the old one, and for a variety of other reasons. There are many such cases in the anecdotal newspaper record. They are pretty easy to find if one takes the time to look. There's Donyea Jones of Seattle, for example, who was shot by his wife in the back of the head (not a case of imminent fear) in front of the children and then was dragged out of the house and set on fire. (Coincidentally, this Seattle murder occurred during October, National Domestic Violence Awareness Month.) However, neither the Seattle newspaper or any domestic violence advocates in Seattle pointed to this case as an example. The murder of famous comedian Phil Hartman by his wife is another case where the news media does not mention the words "domestic violence"—or does not label it as such—when it happens to a man.

Regardless of the anecdotal evidence, Dr. Mann's analysis and other analyses show that a different conclusion can be drawn from the same set of data that Van Wormer cites. The resources for women (shelters and crisis lines) do seem to be saving men's lives, which should only lead us to establish the same types of resources for men, so more women's lives can be saved. To put it another way, shelters and crisis lines offer an opportunity for someone to "cool off" (along with filling other needs). There's a place to go and someone neutral (nonfamily or friend) to talk to. Crisis lines and shelters, legal system advocates, and other helping systems provide an essential mechanism that aid in defusing a family violence situation. Good batterer intervention programs available to men (but not very often to women) may also be helpful. Thus, it is little wonder that the rate of women murdering their spouses has fallen, while the rate of men doing the same to women has remained constant.

The data demonstrate that a wife has a 25 percent greater chance of being killed by her husband than a husband has of being killed by his wife. The statistical figures are less than the percentages most commonly assumed by the popular news media or the general public. As has been the case in previous surveys, women kill their children more often than fathers do (55 percent versus 45 percent). Murder of a child by a parent amounted to 21 percent of all family homicides.[50]

It is well known—but often neglected by policymakers—that men are nearly twice as likely as women to be victims of all types of violent crime and are three times more likely to be murder victims.

Another way of viewing violent female intimate crime is to study the number of prison inmates. The Bureau of Justice Statistics reports: "Women serving a sentence for a violent offense were about twice as likely as their male counterparts to have committed their offense against someone close to them. . . . Women in prison for homicide were almost twice as likely to have killed an intimate (husband, ex-husband, or boyfriend) as a relative like a parent or a sibling" (see Table 1.5).[51]

Coramae Richey Mann, a criminologist at Florida State University, examined nearly 300 female perpetrator homicide cases in six of the largest cities in the United States and published her results in *Justice Quarterly*. Out of the 300, she looked at 145 cleared homicide cases where the arrested woman killed a person who was, or once had been, a live-in lover. While the rate changed in the

Table 1.5
Relationship of Violent Offenders to Their Victims by Gender

Relationship of Victim	Females Who Kill	Males Who Kill
Intimate	19.9%	6.8%
Relative	15.9%	9.6%

years the research went on, about half of all the female homicides occurred in domestic situations.[52]

Common-law marriages and lover relationships had about a 10 percent greater incidence of murder than a legally married status. Of the victims, 3.4 percent were current or former lesbian lovers of the female homicide offender. The remainder were male. About 30 percent of the women who killed their domestic partners had a previous violent arrest record. Furthermore, 70 percent killed their victims when they were drunk, helpless (bound), or asleep. Nearly 60 percent preplanned the killing. Realizing the potentially controversial nature of these findings, Mann devoted a significant portion of her article to the issue of self-defense as a justification for these homicides:

> Previous studies emphasize the self-defense aspect of female homicide cases and suggest that the "helpless little woman" in an altercation in which she is at a physical disadvantage kills the "bullying big man," who has a history of battering her. Women who killed in domestic encounters provide no exception to this scenario and, in fact, denied responsibility for the killing (51.8%) more frequently than non-domestic female killers (48.2%). Although they denied responsibility for the slaying, and attributed it to self-defense or some other cause…in-depth readings of the case files had, however, indicated the contrary possibility that these women were the victors in the domestic fight.
>
> The battered woman syndrome, when used as a rationale for self-defense in a homicide case, suggests that the act was reasonable and necessary because the offender "reasonably believed she was in imminent danger of serious bodily harm or death and the force she used was necessary to avoid that danger.…In addition to the individual case analysis, several other indicators suggest that the battered woman syndrome, although not to be rejected, is not necessarily relevant in many of the domestic homicides studied. First, the majority of the offenders were single and (at least theoretically), could have left the abuser, particularly because they did not appear to reflect the "learned helplessness" typical of battered women. Second, premeditation of the homicides in more than half of the cases challenges the notion of "reasonableness," particularly the "objective immediacy standard" or the woman's belief that she is in immediate danger. Third, previous arrest

histories suggest that some of these offenders were neither helpless nor afraid of their victims.[53]

Another study of women incarcerated for spouse killings found that 60 percent did not report they were the victims of chronic physical abuse.[54] Mann, in an interview, was even more emphatic about these offenders. Basically, she thinks that violent behavior is just that and can rarely be "excused." Her study certainly contradicts a number of commonly held assumptions about female killers in domestic violence cases. She also cautions that DOJ figures may not be giving the complete story:

> Women throughout history have been known to often use poison as a means to carry out a murder. We don't know the level of hidden homicide by women who use poison on their mates, since this method is often undetected; hence, there would be no arrest. Also, the justice system has a history of chivalry and paternalism toward women. Certainly, there are many examples where a man is charged with homicide, while a woman committing a similar act is charged with a lesser offense.[55]

In its prison survey, the DOJ also found a different standard of sentencing for women: "For each category of offense, women received shorter average maximum sentences than men. For property offenses, female prisoners had a mean sentence 42 months shorter than men; for drug offenses, 18 months shorter; and for violent offenses, 39 months shorter." [56]

Mann states that many female murderers who kill their spouses do not get charged with first-degree murder, nor even get recorded in the DOJ statistics, because they hire or persuade a man to do the killing for them. In the DOJ statistics, a contract killing gets registered not as a woman killing her spouse but as a multiple offender homicide. It is important, however, to remember that the overwhelming majority of domestic violence incidences do not result in death or even in severe injury.

PITFALLS OF A FOCUS ON INJURIES

Restraining and protective orders (in most jurisdictions) do not require an observable injury before they are issued; they usually require only an assertion or demonstration of the threat of violence and that there has been violence in the past year, even if that violence did not result in serious injury. If the only focus was on injury-producing violence, the entire system of issuing such court orders would have to be changed, and indeed as we will discuss later, there are needed changes in this part of the system, but that does not mean ignoring credible threats. Most police departments do not require an observable injury in order for someone to be arrested. An arrest can be made solely on the basis of the threat of an attack. Society would understandably not want to return to the days when a woman had to be severely and recently injured before she could get her mate arrested or restrained.

Those who maintain that violence by wives is of little or no concern would have to dramatically revise the rationale for providing services to battered women if only injury-producing assaults were measured. If advocates for battered women had to limit their numbers to the 188,000 women a year who are assaulted with severe injury-producing results (as Straus estimates), the totality of the problem would be underestimated. Use of this figure alone would certainly hamper public education and funding for services.

Use of only the DOJ's National Crime Victim Survey results, which has fluctuated but is trending downward for women at one million to 840,000 intimate violent victimizations against women and 143,000 to 150,000 equally violent male victimizations a year, also underestimates the problem.

THE HIDDEN COSTS OF DOMESTIC VIOLENCE

In an interview with the author, Suzanne Steinmetz says that where we should put resources is one question (see Chapter 5) and that who gets injured the most should not be part of the debate over family violence:

> I believe we should look at all violence as equally bad. It really doesn't matter who ends up with more damage. I get real nervous when we try to say one is more important than the other, or one needs more attention than the other. The bottom line is, in most of these families there are children who are witnessing it, the psychological damage is there. Even when a woman slaps a man, and it doesn't do any physical damage, it is doing damage to his psyche. From my interviews with the women that do this, it's not making her feel very good either. It's an indication that they are out of control. Women do not like to feel out of control. We do not want to be viewed as "hysterical" women. I've had many women tell me how it frightened them, when they realized how they could lose their temper and do this.[57]

Violence in the home, whether committed by women or men, is a serious social problem. The studies show that violence is damaging in a number of ways, not just in terms of physical injury. There is ample evidence that victims of domestic violence suffer grave damage to their self-esteem, thus reducing the opportunity to be productive citizens. Jean, a 41-year-old man, explains: "I didn't have any self-esteem of myself because I took everything personally and I thought what she was saying was true."[58] Domestic violence also contributes to drug and alcohol abuse, mental illness, attempted suicide, and depression.

VIOLENCE AND THE NEXT GENERATION

It is the contribution by women and men to the next generation of violent homes that is the most disturbing aspect of mate abuse. Straus, Gelles, and Steinmetz commented:

> Men who had seen parents physically attack each other were almost three times more likely to hit their own wives....Women whose parents were violent had a much higher rate of hitting their own husbands as compared to the daughters of non-violent parents....In fact, the sons of the most violent parents have a rate of wife-beating 1000 per cent greater than that of the sons of nonviolent parents. The daughters of violent parents have a husband-beating rate that is 600 per cent greater than the daughters who grew up in non-violent households.[59]

Even if children grow up in a family that is nonviolent, they still may not escape domestic violence, since about 10 percent of men and women abusers did not experience a violent family life. It is, however, considerably less likely. Straus, Gelles, and Steinmetz add: "Generally, those who grew up in homes in which parents were violent to each other tended to be violent in their own marriages. It made no difference whether it was the father or mother who was violent, or whether the child was a boy or a girl."[60] Even if we consider only this facet, that violent homes increase the *likelihood* of more violent homes (but not the certainty since the majority of people who experience violence in the home in their childhood years do not go on to have a violent home life in their adult years), there must be concern over violence produced by either gender.

This concern is expressed in more chilling terms by O'Keefer, Brockopp, and Chew who reported findings on teen dating violence in *Social Work*. They reported on studies that found that "an equal number of boys and girls experienced as well as initiated abuse," while their own study found that "overall the girls were violent more frequently than the boys." They confirmed the cycle of abuse in families: "More than half of the students who witnessed their parents being abusive to each other had been involved in an abusive relationship." Even more important, the authors suggest that things will get worse in the next generation: "Unlike older women in violent relationships, teenage girls have less at stake materially and emotionally and may therefore be more willing to take greater risks with their relationships. These findings may also indicate that future generations of women are more likely to participate equally in all aspects of their relationships, including violence." [61]

Their prediction has turned out to be true. In the past 10 years, teenage dating violence surveys have shown an increase in female-initiated violence (although the overall rate between the two genders in the surveys remain roughly equal).

Indeed, some criminal justice researchers believe that given the current trends, female crime will eventually match the male rate for *all* types of crime except for rape and murder. In a study published in *The Journal of Police and Criminal Psychology*, female larceny, for example, is expected to equal the male rate in 2026, burglary in 2237, and assault in 2267, if the present trends continue.[62] Between 1993 and 2002, the female embezzlement arrest rate was actually greater than the number of men arrested on the same charges, the first time in any category that female crime exceeded male crime.

Nationally, according to the FBI's Uniform Crime Report, overall crime fell from 1993 through 2002, and the number of men arrested fell by nearly 6 percent; however, the number of women arrested increased by 14 percent during this time period.

When a woman hits, pushes, or shoves a man—even *if* no physical damage results—when children are present, a clear message is sent to them: Violence is acceptable behavior. Because society is concerned with reducing the incidence of domestic violence in future generations, it must be concerned about violence from both genders, regardless of the extent of physical injuries.

Because the evidence shows that women hit, slap, and are otherwise violent as often as men in domestic situations, an absolute stance should be taken against violence by either gender, not only because of the message it sends to children who observe or become aware of such behavior, but also because it contributes to the incidence of child abuse. Numerous studies show that women commit more acts of child abuse than do men. Certainly, there are factors that help to explain this finding (such as women more often being the primary caretakers of children), but it is clear that one kind of violence prompts other forms of violence. If it is permissible for a woman to slap or hit her mate, is it not then permissible by the same reasoning or standard for her to slap or hit her child?

INCREASING THE CHANCES

Another important reason why advocates for female victims of domestic violence should be concerned about female perpetrators is that when a woman strikes her male partner, she greatly increases her chances of becoming a victim herself. Straus comments:

> Let us assume that most of the assaults by wives...are not intended to, and only rarely cause physical injury....The danger to women is shown by studies that find that minor violence by wives increases the probability of severe assaults by husbands. Sometimes this is immediate and severe retaliation....[A] more indirect and probably more important effect may be that [it]...reinforces the traditional tolerance of assault in marriage.

The moral justification of assault implicit when a woman slaps or throws something at a partner for doing something outrageous reinforces his moral justification for slapping her when she is doing something outrageous, or when she is obstinate, nasty, or "not listening to reason" as he sees it. To the extent this is correct, one of the many steps needed in primary prevention of assaults on wives is for women to forsake even "harmless" attacks on male partners and children. Women must insist on nonviolence from their sisters, just as they rightfully insist on it from men....Although this may seem like "victim blaming," there is an important difference. Recognizing that assaults by wives are one of the many causes of wife beating does not justify such assaults. It is the responsibility of husbands as well as wives to refrain from physical attacks (including retaliation) at home as elsewhere, no matter what the provocation.[63]

GETTING OUT

Economic Restrictions

A common assumption, and one of the most frequently cited rationales for ignoring domestic violence against men, is that women have less of an opportunity to leave a violent relationship than men do. McNeely and Robinson-Simpson comment: "Most people accept the assumption that wives, particularly low-income wives, cannot escape abusive relationships because of financial dependence. Their entrapment is used to explain the desperation of those who resort to spouse killings. Examinations of female spouse abuse victims reveal that low-income women are *more likely* than affluent women to leave domestic arrangements involving spouse abuse."[64]

Dr. Steinmetz also casts doubt on this assumption in "The Battered Husband Syndrome," published in *Victimology:*

> It is always assumed that the husband's greater economic resources could allow him to more easily leave a disruptive marital situation. Not only do men tend to have jobs which provide them with an adequate income, but they have greater access to credit and are not tied to the home because of the children. This perspective rests on erroneous sexist assumptions. Although males, as a group, have considerably more economic security, if the husband leaves the family, he is still responsible for a certain amount of economic support of the family in addition to the cost of a separate residence for himself. Thus, the loss in standard of living is certainly a consideration for any husband who is contemplating a separation....Interviews with abused men suggest that leaving the family home means leaving...the comfortable and familiar, that which is not likely to be reconstructed in a small apartment.[65]

Fear of Losing Contact with Children

An area that inhibits fathers from leaving abusive relationships is their assumption that they will lose custody of their children and be relegated to the role of visiting father, if they are even allowed unblocked visitation. Although figures in the United States show that male custody has increased, women most often win custody in domestic court. Fathers are keenly aware of this fact. Fear of losing day-to-day contact with one's children (perhaps forever) can certainly be viewed as an inhibitor against leaving a violent relationship. This perception by abused fathers is confirmed by Canadian researcher Lesley Gregorash in an unpublished study: She found that in every case where the couples had children together, "The men felt threatened that they might lose custody or access to their children." [66]

Lack of Power

Gregorash says all of the men she studied suffered from low levels of perceived coping efficacy; they felt they had tried every method of dealing with the situation without success. This was expressed in phrases such as "She had total power" and "She had total control." Gregorash says, "The role this perception played was to prevent them from gaining a more equitable balance of power, to keep them, in a sense, in a hostage-captor type relationship."

Those who work with abused women will recognize this perception on the part of the victim as a common one. It should not be surprising, therefore, that it is also a prevalent condition for abused men.

Responsibility for Failure

Leaving the relationship for either gender means the acceptance of failure. Abused men feel a heavy burden in this regard, according to Gregorash: "The perception of being a failure, should the marriage terminate, kept these men from viewing separation or divorce as a possible alternative. Weighing the costs and benefits of all alternatives was, therefore, restricted." Leaving an abusive relationship presents difficulties that are not easily overcome by either gender. There are other assumptions involving gender roles that are not as easily tested.

HARMONY AT ANY PRICE?

Consider this statement by English researcher L. Miller and supported in a report by Canadian Eugen Lupri: "As a culture we are overwhelmingly committed to upholding a unified and harmonious image of family life, but this commitment to maintaining family harmony is still placed squarely on the shoulders of women, not of men."[67] Is this really the case, always? Lupri and others cite the emotional commitment to partners, children, and kin as a "salient factor in the decision to tolerate abuse and to remain in the relationship." A common stereotype is that most men do not want to marry. They give up the freedom of the unattached, they assume much greater financial responsibility, they assume responsibilities in maintaining the home, and they often become the "final resort" in child discipline. Certainly, these and a host of other responsibilities and commitments may act as a disincentive for men to marry, but love, pressure from family, friends, and society, and their mate's own desires often overcome the alleged disincentives.

Do men, then, having accepted these responsibilities and constraints, desire a nonharmonious home any more than women do? It is much more logical to assume that both men and women want a harmonious family life. Therapists routinely report that both men and women know that regardless of whether they themselves were raised in a dysfunctional family, heavy drinking and frequent fighting should not be norms in any family.

Blanket statements that attempt to define gender roles in the family, based on old stereotypes, do both genders a serious disservice. This leads directly to the core of the argument used to ignore or downplay the issue of male spousal abuse as a serious social problem.

PATRIARCHY

Consider this statement: A patriarchal societal structure exists that has as its basis the subjugation of women. Given this structure, women in an abusive relationship have fewer resources than men by which to escape. It is this patriarchy that condones and accepts violence against women. Domestic violence against men should not be placed on a par with domestic violence against women, because the violence against women is a result of a male-dominated society.

This argument is repeated, in one form or another, in virtually all of the books about domestic violence. Historically, one would have had to agree with it. The Napoleonic Code, for example, stated, "Women, like walnut trees, should be beaten every day." Throughout the centuries, women have been buried alive, burned, or tortured for such things as having a miscarriage, even when caused by the husband. It has taken a long time for the right of the man to be absolute lord and master in his home to be questioned and to have legal sanctions put against him for battering his wife, at least in Western countries. It is relevant to note that men who suffered battering by their wives were also subject to public humiliation and censure. Steinmetz reports this historical background:

> The charivari, a post-renaissance custom, was a noisy demonstration intended to shame and humiliate wayward individuals in public. The target

was any behavior considered to be a threat to the patriarchal community social order. Thus in France, a husband who allowed his wife to beat him was made to wear an outlandish outfit, ride backwards around the village on a donkey while holding onto the tail. Beaten husbands among the Britons were strapped to carts and paraded ignominiously through the booing populace.... The fate of these men in 18th century Paris was to kiss a large set of ribboned horns.[68]

Since we are speaking of the historical record here, it should be noted that it is an urban myth that the phrase "rule of thumb" came from a law that said a woman could be beaten with a stick no bigger around than a thumb. No such law has ever existed in any English-speaking country.

Certainly, there are many cases in which a woman still must overcome great obstacles in convincing authorities that she is a battered wife. Men also face similar obstacles.

If the patriarchal system is at the root of wife battering, and not other, more important factors such as upbringing, learned behavior, stress, drinking, and lack of conflict resolution skills, then the situations of men and women are very different, and our response to domestic violence—even in today's world—must be different for the genders. There is considerable hard data now that question this assumption.

"Patriarchy" + Conservative Religion = Wife Abuse?

"Judeo-Christian doctrine, which espoused the inferiority of women and the supremacy of men, gave its stamp of approval to domestic violence," says *Battered Wives* author Del Martin.[69] Although Martin is speaking of the historical record, the modern assumption is that this is still true.

Merlin Brinkerhoff, Elaine Grandin, and Eugen Lupri used the large-scale Canadian survey of family violence mentioned earlier to examine religion, patriarchy, and domestic violence. They report on their findings in the *Journal for the Scientific Study of Religion:*

> Feminists and some social scientists have argued that violence used by men against women in the conjugal relationship reflects male supremacy and a patriarchal order. Much of the rationale for suggesting a relationship between religion and wife abuse stems from the assumption that members of the more fundamentalist groups tend to be more patriarchal.... Some people would posit that continued male dominance will lead to increased family violence.... In the few studies that have explored the role of religious commitment in family violence, church attendance was used as the indicator of religious commitment. The more frequent the attendance, it was assumed, the higher the commitment to the values of the group.... Frequent attendance

at churches with strong values on patriarchy might actually increase spousal violence.... The data provide only limited support for this patriarchy thesis; 28.1% of the [c]onservative Protestants committed violent acts against their intimate partners during the past year. However, contrary to what one might expect from the theoretical rationale, it was not the conservative males but rather the females who were the most abusive toward their mates. Those identifying with no denomination were most violent among males and were the second most abusive among women and in the sample as a whole.... *The prediction based on the patriarchy assumption* (i.e., increased violence with increased attendance) *was not supported.* In fact, the lowest rates of spousal violence were found among those attending church services weekly or more often. [Emphasis added][70]

The results of the research concerning church attendance contradict the patriarchy thesis, which suggests that highly committed conservative Protestant males would be the most violent: "To sum up, neither denomination nor attendance seemed to affect spousal violence. The patriarchy thesis, as related to religion, is thus questionable. Other variables, mainly spousal interaction factors, were found to be the best overall predictors of such physical abuse."

This early study has been replicated by further research in the United States that substantiates the general premise: Male regular church attendees have the same or lower (in most studies) rate of intimate partner abuse than the general population; females have the same or slightly higher (in most studies) rate.

Women versus Women—Where's the Patriarchy?

Another frequently mentioned assumption about domestic violence is that male dominance is a causal factor in producing wife abuse. Stated another way, if society did not condone male dominance, fewer women would be battered. Women who are free of male domestic dominance should then be free of domestic violence.

However, Mann's previously cited study of females who commit homicide found that 3.4 percent were women who killed their lesbian mates or lovers. *Naming the Violence: Speaking Out about Lesbian Battering,* edited by Kerry Lobel for the National Coalition against Domestic Violence Lesbian Task Force, contains a record of abuse between female partners (unfortunately, the book does not provide any data about how often such abuse occurs in lesbian relationships). There is ample testimony from the various writers in the book that such abuse does occur and with more frequency than many in the lesbian or battered women's shelter communities acknowledge. Sue Knollenberg, Brenda Douville, and Nancy Hammond of the Task Force on

Violence in Lesbian Relationships commented on this phenomenon in *Naming the Violence:*

> Many of us saw the absence of services to lesbians within the battered women's movement as an area needing attention.... [A] number of questions surfaced. Did it really happen? Could it be as prevalent as male-female battering? The presence of violence deeply affected our vision of ourselves and our relationships.... We were surprised and saddened by the magnitude of the problem and the severity of the violence.... Many women in the broader battered women's movement are affected by the public acknowledgment of lesbian violence. This acknowledgment forces a deepening of the analysis of sexism and male/female roles as contributors to violence in relationships. To understand violence in lesbian relationships is to challenge and perhaps rework some of these beliefs.[71]

Many of the writers in this book expressed similar views. Another myth that was challenged by informal surveys of lesbian batterers and victims was that the violence was limited only to those influenced by predominantly patriarchal structures into strictly "butch/femme" roles. The surveys and testimony showed otherwise, because feminist lesbians also engaged in domestic violence. Claire Renzetti in her book *Violent Betrayal: Partner Abuse in Lesbian Relationships* finds that lesbians batter each other at about the same rate as couples in heterosexual relationships. Other studies indicate an even higher rate.[72] The NVAWS reported a lower rate among lesbian couples compared to the heterosexual population; however, the results were obtained from fewer than 50 such couples.

Another significant study in this area was published in the *Journal of Sex Research* and found that 12 percent of gay males studied reported being victims of forced sex by current or most recent partners, and 31 percent of lesbians reported forced sex. It is possible that men are more inclined than women to underreport acts of sexual violence, but the higher than two-to-one ratio of lesbians reporting violent sexual acts by their partners versus gay men counters the common and repeated assertions of domestic violence being the progeny of male patriarchy (see Figure 1.6).

The contributors to *Naming the Violence: Speaking Out about Lesbian Battering* made it clear that they feared the revelations might harm the battered women's movement. This was certainly not their purpose, nor is it the intent of this book.

The horrifying stories from the Middle East of women being stoned to death because they were raped and other kinds of punishments and restrictions against women in many societies should lead us to the conclusion that

Figure 1.6
Gay and Lesbian Violent/Forced Sex Acts

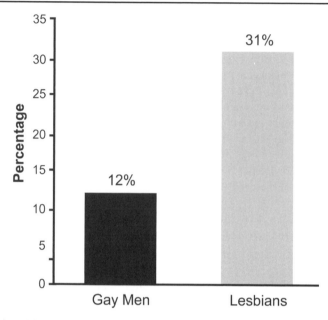

Note: Adapted from C. K. Waterman, L. T. Dawson, and M. J. Bolgna, "Sexual Coercion in Gay Male and Lesbian Relationships: Predictors and Implications for Support Services," *Journal of Sex Research* 26 (1989): 118–124.

patriarchy in its many forms is real in underdeveloped countries and indeed continues to be present in the West. Societal structures do have an influence and what is allowed or not allowed by law and society obviously has an effect on what happens. On the other hand, the Western world is only just beginning to have some understanding of Middle Eastern society. As usual, not all is at it seems. I recall a remarkable conversation with an American flight attendant and "helper" to a wealthy Arab sheik with a harem. The real power in the structure outside the home, basically dealing with those outside the family unit, clearly resided with the sheik. On the other hand, regarding nearly all aspects of home and family life including how money was spent on nonbusiness-related items, the woman said that all power clearly resided with the first wife and not the man.

The evidence is clear. When we paint with too broad a brush, and assume that problems within every male/female/gay/lesbian/transgendered relationship can be blamed on societal structures, we obscure individual circumstances. The most important causal factors for abuse are more complex than patriarchy and are primarily related to circumstances in the family of origin and individuals choosing to be violent. It is not, however, out of place to make a claim that men and women differ in biological makeup. The question then becomes: Are men "naturally" more aggressive than women, and would that lead to more domestic violence perpetrators who are male?

A DIFFERENCE IN THE WIRING?

It would take another book (perhaps several) to attempt to answer this question. Researchers have, however, measured conditioned, aggressive tendencies of men and women in mainly laboratory settings. One of the most comprehensive efforts to examine a large mass of this literature was published in the *Psychological Bulletin* and titled "Are Women Always Less Aggressive Than Men? A Review of the Experimental Literature." Authors Ann Frodi, Jacqueline Macaulay, and Pauline Ropert-Thome examined 72 studies that measured human aggressive behavior. They also looked at 80 books and journals generally referring to aggression. Their conclusion seems to contradict the basic assumption about the differences between men and women:

> The commonly held [belief] that men are almost always more physically aggressive than women and that women display more indirect or displaced aggression [is] not supported.... There is also evidence in the experimental literature, which we review, that women are often as openly hostile and as directly aggressive as men, and occasionally more so.... When we turned to studies of one or another single aggressive response, we did not find that women showed consistently lower tendencies than men to be physically aggressive... or verbally aggressive, whether in a face-to-face situation or not.

The researchers found that aggression and aggressive tendencies of both genders could be changed:

> If sex differences were due to differences in the wiring, it would not seem likely that mere situational or attitudinal changes could erase them. We would argue that behavior is largely shaped by social forces and that these may exaggerate or minimize whatever biological differences may exist.[73]

If it is true that social forces are more important than biological forces when it comes to aggression, it is not surprising that a three-year observational recording of high school students in El Camino, California, found that, among the students observed, it is more socially acceptable for girls to hit boys than vice versa. The observing teacher found that girls hit boys at a 20-to-1 ratio, or 95 percent more often.[74]

How do women feel about the idea that men are "naturally" more aggressive than women? Do they believe this? Is it socially acceptable for a woman to beat up a man?

One thousand women, ages 18 to 25, were questioned by BKG Youth Inc., and the results were published in *Esquire* magazine. Respondents were asked if they agreed or disagreed with the statement, "Men are assertive and dominant, while women are more nurturing and submissive." Sixty-eight percent disagreed with this statement, and 30 percent agreed. Another question was, "If, for one day only, you had the power to beat up any man, how many men would you beat up?" Only 28 percent said they would not choose to beat up any man, 24 percent gave no answer, and the remainder were almost equally divided in choosing to beat up from one to 10 men.[75]

ABC Primetime broadcast a segment in which two male and female actors were hired to pretend partner violence in a public park, that of the woman pounding her boyfriend with a rolled-up newspaper. They photographed the reactions of passers-by. A majority paused, but only one person tried to intervene in a mild manner. One woman, though, was caught on camera doing a pumped-fist "atta-woman" salute.

The relatively primitive state of scientific understanding of biological differences between men and women indicates there will continue to be debate for a long time over just how much a difference there is and of what that difference consists. Surprising things do keep happening; for instance, an annual meeting of the Endocrine Society produced papers contending that a deficiency of the "male" hormone testosterone was more likely to produce aggressive behavior, not high levels of the androgen. Another study presented findings that estrogen, the "female" hormone, was a source of aggressive tendencies.[76]

Perhaps the only safe assumption we can make about "innate" or "biological" differences between the sexes is that it is safest not to make assumptions. This is a good guide to behaviors and our attitudes toward those behaviors in the world outside the laboratory as well.

SEXISM HURTS EVERYBODY

Shelters and other service providers that fail to recognize that men can also be victims of abuse discriminate against women. Male perpetrators get a lot of assistance; for example, they are commonly referred to batterer intervention programs. Female perpetrators, by not being recognized as such, often fail to get assistance, and they and their families do not receive needed intervention in a timely fashion.

Are men and women still stuck in the old patterns of a "woman's place" and a "man's place" in the Western world? Of course! Must there be a continuing struggle to overcome male chauvinism and the subjugation of women all over the world? Certainly.

The question of who is the "most important" victim is a debate, however, that serves only to detract from providing effective and helpful services for both genders that must have as their goal changing behaviors. Through the hard work of the women's movement, things have changed for the better in many areas for both genders and for battered women in particular. Equality, not victimology, should remain the hallmark of this movement. Ignoring or dismissing the very real needs of the male subjected to domestic abuse contributes to a cycle of family abuse for the next generation. It contributes to gay and lesbian and transgendered victims and perpetrators getting little attention. It does the female heterosexual perpetrator, or the woman locked into a mutual combat role with a male, no good.

Ellen Pence is a founder of the Domestic Abuse Intervention Project in Duluth, Minnesota, and she is a national leader in the battered women's movement. She told a writer for the *New York Times,* "Domestic violence against men is just not a social problem."[77]

The general movement sparked by the first edition of this book resulted in these comments (along with mine) in a nationally distributed Associated Press feature article: "Do women batter? Sure, but not very often," says Bonnie Campbell, who headed the federal Violence Against Women office under President Clinton. "The more success we have as a society in highlighting violence against women, the more of a backlash we get," she said. "I view a lot of this talk about battered men as a significant part of the backlash." Rita Smith, executive director of the National Coalition Against Domestic Violence, adds, "Men choose violence much more often than women; that's a reality that it would be dangerous for the police to ignore." Smith also told the Associated Press reporter that some of the impetus behind the battered-men's movement comes from men who have been abusers themselves. The president of the National Organization for Women, Patricia Ireland, said that she can empathize with men who are victimized. "If I were a guy who'd been battered and nobody seemed to care, I'd probably have some deep anger myself," she said. "You are injured. You are, culturally, an object of ridicule. The support services are harder to find." But, Ireland told the Associated Press, women are "overwhelmingly" the most frequent victims of domestic violence. She said the legitimate concerns of battered men "have been hijacked by anti-feminist advocates and policy-makers for their own political purposes."[78]

Interestingly enough, the NVAWS was seen as an attempt by feminist advocates as a better survey, which would contradict the other scientific surveys stating that female intimate partner perpetration was indeed a significant social problem, and that it did occur with at least nearly the frequency of male violence. The finding that 36 percent of all the victims of severe violence were male, at a rate of 885,000 a year, must not have set too well with this group.

While making the case for equality of services and recognition, however, it is not my intention to set up a males-versus-females battle over who should receive greater attention or more social services. How this might be accomplished with fairness, sanity, without political agendas of any stripe, and better attention to science and demonstrable results is explored in detail in the final chapter.

To reduce domestic violence, we must develop a whole-family approach based on education and coordination of efforts. It is not "victim blaming" to understand that both men and women can, and most often do, contribute to this most significant societal problem. It is also particularly important to realize that "one size does not fit all," that the violence ranges from severe frequent battering and verbal abuse (Lincoln) to minor perhaps one-time incidents (Clinton). To fully appreciate what happens in relationships with males as the primary victims of physical attack, it is helpful to hear directly from those who have experienced it. This testimony is the focus of the next chapter. We will also hear from those who have closely studied these men.

Chapter 2

Telling Their Stories:
Men Speak Out

Before we hear some abused men's personal stories, I will briefly discuss how the following interviews were conducted.

All the names, unless, specifically noted, have been changed. About 30 victims from the western United States were interviewed, and a representative sample of these interviews is presented here. Locations, where necessary to mention, were changed or generalized. Identity protection was sometimes necessary to obtain the interview because some of the men feared retribution. Remaining anonymous allowed these men to speak more freely. Occupations and other identifying characteristics were changed but kept in general context. In one case, the actual names of the people involved were used because the information came from a public source. Since the first publication of this book, some men have suggested that their real names could be used instead of being anonymous, and indeed, one man appeared with me on a national cable television network show and in another case, one man has become a notable spokesperson for the issue, even giving successful seminars on domestic violence to the U.S. Armed Services and many others. In fairness to everyone, however, I've let the interview names stand as they were.

In some instances, the story of the abused man is given as a general narrative with only slight editing—in cases where the flow of the interview lent itself well to simply repeating what he had to say. In other cases, a question-and-answer type of interview is used because it more clearly demonstrates how the men were feeling, or how they responded to a particular question was significant.

In providing general themes for the men's stories, I have relied heavily on both the interviews conducted with abused men in a thesis by Canadian Leslie Gregorash and in Malcolm George's report to Parliament in England. The Sacramento, California, support group reports provided by Curt Engbritson were also used in finding some cohesion of views.[1]

Since the first publication of this book, the number of abused men I have talked to or interviewed or others have, and reported their findings to me, has substantially increased. I have not kept an exact count, but it most likely approaches several hundred men. In addition, I have heard from many others who have worked closely in some official capacity with such men. They agree that, despite our increasing awareness and the greater numbers of men interviewed either on the record or off, not much as changed for the general experience since the first publication of this book.

NATURE OF THE ABUSE

A focus on injury-producing results of domestic violence may distract from other consequences, as Steinmetz pointed out in the previous chapter. It is important, however, to demonstrate the range of the perpetrator's rage and its effect on the victim. Physical attacks do raise the level of domestic abuse, adding to, and often increasing, psychological damage.

Before exploring the effects of the abuse, therefore, we need to hear what happened in the victim's own words. What follows is a cross section of various kinds of attacks. Of the men I have interviewed, only a few are represented in this section. These represent a range of physical acts, but my total small sample did conform to expectations from national surveys; that is, most involved minor violence (slapping, pushing, grabbing, shoving, and/or throwing things) rather than serious violence (hitting, kicking, using a weapon, and/or threatening with a weapon).

One of the most common methods of attack reported by the men I interviewed was their mates' habit of throwing at them anything that was at hand. According to a study of 328 married couples published in *the Journal of Marriage and the Family*, "Women were significantly more likely to throw an object, slap, kick/bite/hit with fist, and hit with an object."[2] The experiences presented here come as no surprise.

Throwing Things

Tim S. is a 25-year-old college student who lived with his girlfriend Mary for two years. He has no children.

> She threw things, anything that was handy, usually glass things, things that were breakable. I mean, we went through a lot of dishes and glasses. When

I got mad, I would throw things, too, but not at her, like she did me. After these arguments, we would make up, and she would say how sorry she was, then want to make love.

Other men interviewed told similar stories. Some of the objects thrown included a heavy padlock (while holding a child—it missed); a crystal lamp (requiring stitches to the forehead); a hammer (it missed); and knives (missing in one case, connecting in another and requiring stitches).

Richard C. is 48 years old and makes an upper-income living in financial services. He married Janet C. when he was 28, and the marriage lasted 14 years. It was a second marriage for both partners. They shared their home with six adopted children and two children from her former marriage. In the course of their years together, there were 50 to 60 physical attacks, he said. Most occurred when she had been drinking:

> Actually, things began before we got married. She would lose her temper and throw things at me. The first time, I was walking down the hall (after I told her she shouldn't give up on her children, who were in foster care at the time), and a set of keys hit me in the back of the head. That was the first thing she did to me, but before that, there was a situation where her father had to pull her and her mother apart when they were fighting on the floor.
>
> A lot of times, I would be working on some papers and there would be a coffee cup there, and she would intentionally spill the coffee; she went from that to throwing the coffee, and then throwing the cup and the coffee. She would throw hot scalding coffee in my face. It was a gradual thing that built over a three-year period, until it got to the point where she would physically strike me.
>
> I had never seen physical abuse between my parents, I had never had physical abuse by my parents, and to be marrying into something with the same socioeconomic status and finding out that…whoa, I had a wolverine here that would go out of control…, that's why it was so hard for me. Afterwards, she would cry and beg forgiveness. But she had done damage. Not only emotionally and psychologically but physically.
>
> She would reach up and grab my glasses (these were the old wire-rim days), and she could twist these into a pretzel. I got into the habit of keeping a spare pair in the car. She would hit me with things. One time we had an argument, and I decided to let her go into the bedroom and let her settle down, so I went to sleep on the couch. About an hour later, I was awakened with a terrible pain on my forehead. She had taken one of my cowboy boots and, with the heel, whacked me in the forehead.

Sleep Deprivation and Attacks

Apparently attacks on abused men such as Richard C. describes are not uncommon. Malcolm George interviewed a number of abused men in England

and found that attacks during sleep periods were reported fairly often.[3] Abused boyfriend Tim S. related one such incident to me: "One time, I got woken up to her pounding real hard with her fists on my head. She said she had a dream that I was cheating on her."

As previously noted, criminologist Coramae Mann found that a significant number of women who kill their mates do so while they are helpless, including being asleep. Curt Engbritson says one of the men in his support group had a split sternum caused by a spouse who had hit him with doubled fists in the chest while he was asleep.

One of the most common techniques for torturing prisoners is sleep deprivation. Studies have shown that it does not take long before a human, being deprived of sleep, becomes disoriented and confused. George says that this subject was brought up "pretty regularly" in his interviews with male victims:

> The women would successfully sleep deprive the man. The man had a job to hold down and he had to go to work. Quite often the women had jobs as well. But if they didn't, or needed less sleep normally than their partner, or could more easily make up their own sleep time lost, because of their part-time job, they would successfully sleep deprive the man. Over a period of months, in which a man say, would usually require eight hours of sleep, but was only allowed four hours, he would become so disoriented that he was literally putty in her hands.

While the samples may be small, there seems to be a pattern that an abusive woman can successfully use methods to overcome her lack of physical stature when attacking her mate.

There are men I have talked with who before going to sleep each night, take care to hide the knives.

Groin Attacks

The most horrifying aspect of domestic violence is when a man intentionally strikes the belly of a pregnant woman, actions that have been documented in many instances. Obviously, no equivalent exists for male victims; however, George found it is a common tactic for female perpetrators to hit or, more commonly, kick their partners in the testicles. A number of the victims I interviewed also reported this, but most reported an attempt rather than an actual blow. Some reported that their partners would threaten this, then say that it was only a humorous threat. It still made the men nervous. George reports one case in which the victim was barricaded inside his home by his wife, who put furniture in front of the door, then hit him on the chest and kicked him in the groin.

Richard C. says this was a common pattern for his wife:

She would physically attack me, tear the glasses off, kick me in the testicles five, six, seven times....You couldn't control her. A couple of times, I would wrestle her to the ground, pin her arms around her, and wrap my legs around her, and tell her to calm down, calm down. She'd say "O.K. I'm calm now, I'm under control now." And you let her go, and she'd be right back at you, doing it again.

Biting

Richard C. says he had one of his children telephone his wife's psychologist while he was holding her down: "[The child] hears this yeow and says, 'What happened?' I say, 'She just bit me in the ass.' I thought I had her pinned down, but she wriggled free and got me."

Mark K. is married to Joan K. Their divorce was still pending at the time of the interview. They have one child, a girl, who is three years old. Mark works all shifts, usually swing, at a warehouse. Joan is a homemaker. He says his wife would frequently kick, scratch, hit, and throw things:

Tell me about the time you were most seriously hurt.

I had seen my lawyer about two weeks before this happened. I was thinking seriously about a divorce. I got home at about ten o'clock at night, and no one was there. I figured she had gone to the neighbors, so I asked them, and they told me that she and a friend had gone to a store. But, I knew that store closed at ten, so I went into this tavern right next to it. She was in there, pretty smashed. I went in there and bought a beer right over the top of her head, and she didn't even know I was there. She was going to leave with some of her girlfriends. I told her it was time to go home, and she didn't want to come with me. I did persuade her to come with me finally and she got into the truck. We got over to the baby-sitter's house and picked up [our child], but my wife didn't want to leave with me. She was starting one of her fits again.

I said O.K....she could stay there, the [Smiths] are friends as well as baby-sitters, but I told her the baby would have to come with me. When she gets drunk, she just takes off with the baby. She had, a bunch of times, gone walking in pitch-dark along the river road, staggering drunk, with the kid. I wouldn't know where she was, or anything. So, I wasn't going to let that happen again, so I just grabbed her and the kid and put them in the truck. I just restrained her. I drove around for about an hour, because if I stopped, I knew that she would just get out and start walking. Who knows where. I got her home, and sure enough, she took the baby and started to take off. I got the baby away from her, and she ran up from behind and bit me on the shoulder and once on the chest. I could have dropped the baby because of what she was doing.

Did you go to the hospital?

No, I didn't. The bites were pretty deep, though; I still have scars that don't look like they are ever going away. It really did hurt a lot. I did have [my lawyer] take pictures.

Domestic violence incidents related by the men interviewed cannot be viewed in isolation by type of attack. Most often, two or more events are combined. For example, one man described an incident in which he was sleeping, was hit over the head with a beer bottle, and then was bitten in the leg.

Alcohol and Weapon Use

Mark K. believed that his wife's drinking was directly associated with her violent acts. In the case of Marvin T., his wife's drinking was also involved and escalated into weapon use.

Marvin was married to his alcoholic wife for seven years. She was often verbally abusive when she was drinking. They argued frequently. When they met, they were both heavy drinkers. Five and a half years after they got married, Marvin became involved in a church that his wife did not attend. With the help of the minister and church members, as well as Alcoholics Anonymous, he admitted his problem with alcohol and stopped drinking.

She did not stop. He became less argumentative, but the battles between them grew more intense and her verbal abuse increased, especially when he urged her to examine her drinking habits. The verbal abuse began to change into physical assaults. She began pushing and shoving him, and several times she took swings at him. He felt this was something he could handle by dodging the blows or warding them off with his arms or just leaving home for a while. One night, it became something he could not handle:

> We lived in a trailer. When I got home, I could tell she'd been drinking really hard, by the bottles laying around and the way she acted. She started yelling at me, and not really making much sense. I basically told her to go fuck off and shut up. I mean, in a trailer court, the neighbors can hear a lot. I guess that's who did call the cops eventually.
>
> I'm kind of tall and not really heavy, so I would guess that she outweighed me by a good twenty pounds or more. Well, we had this door with a glass top part and screen bottom. She just gave me a big shove, and bang into the top part of the door I went with my arm, and the glass broke. I didn't get caught in the neck, thank God, but I did get some cuts and was bleeding. But I guess

that wasn't enough for her. I was yelling pretty good at her, and she ran into the kitchen, which was really just a couple of steps, and got out this steak knife and started stabbing me, overhand, and coming down hard. I was for getting the hell out of there, I tell you!

I know she got me seven times because of what they said later at the emergency ward; luckily, the stab wounds were not that deep, and only a couple needed stitches, five stitches for one, and three or four for another. The rest, they just cleaned and bandaged.

You won't believe this part! Sure, her drinking and me stopping was a big part of it, but I also knew that she had been having an affair. Now you gotta realize that this is a small town we lived in. So, I pretty much knew for sure who it was, and it was one of the local cops.

Guess who shows up at this fight? Right, the cop she'd been screwing. Well, guess who gets arrested? Yep, me. Not only that, the son-of-a-bitch handcuffs me, puts me in the back of the squad car, and says when we get out of the [trailer] court that I've been uncooperative and resistant to arrest! He was real calm and matter-of-fact. He pulls over where it's dark, gets out this big flashlight and punches me in the ribs with it four or five times, and pops me on the head too, all the while telling me what an asshole I am. He did take me to the emergency room. I got a little cleaned up and got my stitches and stuff, and then I was put in jail.

When I got out, I had had enough. I started on the divorce. I was just glad we didn't have any kids.

Weapon Use after Escaping

It is often assumed that men, once they leave the abusive relationship, are not in as much danger as women of being stalked, tracked down, or abused again. The research is incomplete, even though the National Violence Against Women Survey did measure stalking. Police reports contain inadequate data sources since they cannot track the unreported incidents nor the cases in which people other than the spouse are sent to harm men who leave. Such cases are recorded as multiple offender incidents and not as cases of domestic violence.

In any event, multiple offender "track down" cases, and even cases in which the former spouse uses a weapon to attack or kill her partner, are not often labeled as examples of domestic violence in the news media when the victim is male. A case in point is that of Steven and Marcia Moskowitz. The couple were prominent community members in Portland, Oregon, and had been married for 16 years. She worked for the city planning bureau, had also been a social worker, and later became an organizer for the Oregon Nurses Association. He served as deputy city attorney, joined the mayor's staff, and then became a senior partner in a prominent private practice law firm. Both were well respected and very active in political and social affairs. They had two children, a boy from her previous marriage and a girl who was 11 when they separated.

In January 1992, Steven moved out of the house. In October of that year, Marcia shot Steven five times, repeatedly pulling the trigger until the gun was empty. Steven spent two months in the hospital; except for a severely hampered walk, he miraculously recovered.

The attempted murder sent a shock wave through the upper echelons of the Portland community. Friends of Marcia immediately suspected, and commented to the press, that she must have been a victim of abuse for her to have done something like this. Steven has consistently refused all comment to the press. After the trial, Marcia told *The Oregonian,* a daily newspaper: "It was very hard for me to imagine where I could end up going. My choices felt like they were narrowed down. I just felt no sense of future."[4] She bought a .22 caliber pistol and learned how to shoot it.

Both she and Steven used a local exercise club. Steven had met his new girlfriend at the same club. One time, Marcia saw the woman there and hit her. In a letter to a friend, Marcia said it made her feel good to hit the woman. Marcia thought that Steven had agreed to stay away from the club; then she learned that he planned to attend a staff performance one night. She called him three times on his answering machine, screaming that he had no right to interfere in her space. But she felt the messages weren't enough: "I had to face him and make him listen to me."

She went to his apartment, and Steven let her in. She started to talk about him going to the club, and he said things were changing and this was something she was going to have to get used to. She pulled the gun out. According to her, she said, "I just want you to be quiet and listen to what I have to say." She claimed Steven "[s]ighed, rolled his eyes and said 'Oh right, Marcia, I suppose you're going to shoot me.'" She felt he was brushing her off, "like a little fly."

According to Steven's version in police reports, he told her she could have all the property in the divorce, that she could "have it all." She replied, "You bet I can," and began shooting. Marcia says he cursed her and took one step toward her, and he was really angry. "I knew if he took the gun away from me, he could hurt me. Would he have shot me? I don't think so. I think I know that much.... So the first shot was fired. The way I remember it is like closing my eyes and pulling the trigger." He started moving away down a hallway outside the apartment and yelling to another tenant to call 911. "At that point, I'm just shooting madly. It's more like I'm watching myself than feeling it. But I'm aiming down at his legs. I saw somebody down at the end of hall and part of my mind was saying, 'Oh my God, what are you doing? This is just too bizarre.' And then the gun was empty." Steven was wounded in the legs, and a bullet fragment had also lodged near his heart; out of the total six wounds, most were in the chest and abdomen.

Marcia was charged with attempted murder and first-degree assault. During bail hearings, defense attorneys contended that she was not an escape risk, and she consented to electronic monitoring. She was released on bail. The prosecuting attorney said that Steven was concerned that Marcia "will hunt him down and finish the job she started." At the bail hearing, her defense attorney said that he would show that Marcia had been the victim of increasingly severe violence. The prosecutors placed in evidence letters and other diary writings that had been sent to Steven. Prosecutor Helen Smith said that Marcia's writings show that Steven Moskowitz was a kind and generous husband who was perhaps too passive to suit Marcia. She noted that Marcia wrote of having to "kick him in the butt to get him going." There was no trial. Instead, Marcia pleaded no contest. She apologized to the court: "What I did was not decent or justified or right. I am profoundly sorry for my actions."

The prosecutor reminded the court that Marcia had stood over Steven and continued to pull the trigger even after the gun was empty, while he lay bleeding on the floor. Marcia was given a shortened two-year prison term. The judge noted that it was Steven's plea before the court that resulted in the reduced term. Tearfully, Steven said, "The person I think about most in all of this is our daughter. I don't think it would serve her welfare to have a protracted trial in this matter. I speak to you today more as a father than as a victim; my daughter needs her mother." Steven was later granted custody, but Marcia was given extensive visitation rights.

In prison, Marcia told the newspaper: "I know what I did was wrong. I am so glad Steven didn't die....I know I didn't intend to shoot him when I went to his apartment. I don't want to legitimize in any way what I did. I guess I am finally coming to the point where I am saying, 'Whoa, this wasn't all my fault.' It took two people to make something like this happen."

Despite the original widespread publicity surrounding this case, the words *domestic violence* were never used in subsequent news reports about the trial or Steven Moskowitz's recovery. These words were only used when friends of Marcia Moskowitz were initially interviewed about their suspicions. When it became apparent that he was the victim, not her, the newspaper no longer reported it as a case of "domestic violence."

We will explore in greater detail the role of the news media and the male victim in Chapter 4. The lack of media and social recognition of the male victim does play a significant role in how these men view themselves, whether they are the victims of severe attacks or minor ones.

BEWILDERED MEN'S REPONSES TO ABUSE

It does not seem to matter what kind of abuse the male partner experiences. Male victims who have been interviewed seem to share a common outcome: They are, indeed, bewildered. For them, there are no rules as to how they should act or respond. They seem to be searching for a set of guidelines that do not exist. They want to apply logic to an illogical situation. Time after time, men in their stories would ask, "What was I supposed to do?" It is a plea for some direction.

Curt Engbritson coordinated one of the few support groups in the United States for battered men. The group operated out of the Sacramento (California) Men's Center. Usually about 6 to 10 men participated in each group. Engbritson agreed that bewilderment was a primary emotion for these men, which led to frustration:

> They know when there is going to be an escalation into violence since, by the time they get into the group, it's not an isolated incident. They don't know how to stop it. They don't seem to think of any other recourse but to stay in the thick of it—the argument that was going on. So, they lacked the skills to deal with stopping the argument.

Not knowing what else to do, many withdraw. One man was married for 25 years to a woman who was constantly verbally abusive. He withdrew, would hide behind a newspaper, but this only made her even more angry, and it would sometimes escalate into physical abuse. He was a quiet type, and she was a volatile type. They also came from different ethnic and national backgrounds, which contributed to the conflict. Because the men all say they can't or won't hit a woman, even though they are being hit or having things thrown at them, they don't know what their response should be, so the sense of frustration mounts.

For some men, any area that does not have clearly defined rules brings uneasiness. What are the rules for a man who is, or has been, struck or seriously assaulted by his mate? Does he hit back? No. Not only is it wrong; he might seriously injure her, and even in a case of self-defense, he might be arrested. Many men do respond with violence of their own (as we learned in Chapter 1, about 50 percent of all domestic violence is mutual), but many others do not hit back.

Not Hitting Back

Joe S. explains:

> Things started out pretty good, the first couple of years. Then, I don't know, she slowly changed. I mean, she always had a temper, but then we got into

some money problems, and it got worse. She would get mad, and it would just escalate all out of proportion. She'd start hitting. She'd slap at my face, and then keep slapping and trying to scratch me. I'd put up my arms or just grab and hold her hands. I never hit her back. I was just taught that you never hit a woman.

Jeff W. adds:

It's almost like it was ingrained in me, from the time I was a little kid. You don't hit girls, you just don't. I would hold her arms, I guess pretty tightly in the heat of the moment. She did get some finger mark bruises on her arms once, but what was I supposed to do, just let her keep hitting me? Still, I couldn't hit back. The first time it happened, I was just shocked and figured it was a onetime thing. It was just one slap, and I blocked it, and that was the end of it, or so I thought.

Steve J. was married for 12 years. He came to my attention by way of his stepdaughter. She had watched his abuse at the hands of her mother for many years and thought he was someone I should interview. She confirmed the lack of retaliation on his part. He is a well-paid professional architect. He describes the family income as upper middle class. I talked with him just six months after he had left the relationship. At first, he said he might have trouble recalling all that had happened; since leaving he had "blocked out" things in an attempt to put the painful memories behind him:

If she got really irate about something, she would come over to me and start pushing and slapping. She would just push, sometimes enough to slam me into a wall.

Steve said his wife would also frequently throw glass objects and sometimes got pushy in public.

What was your reaction when she pushed you, in public or in private?

I usually clammed up. I was good at that. I pretty much backed off. I got the feeling that she would not do it more than once, so I would just back off out of her reach. I would go into my office [in his home] or someplace other than where she was.

Were you shocked by what she did?

At first, I was shocked by her violence. Or, maybe surprised. But towards the end, I guess I wasn't surprised as much.

Did you ever hit her?

No, I'm not that type of person. I don't hit women. I don't hit really any-body. I'm not a physical person like that. I don't react to physical violence in kind, never have. I might hit a man back, but because she's a woman... I just don't think it's proper.

What makes it not proper? What in your background told you that it wasn't proper?

I guess family and environment, what you learned in school about boys not hitting girls—that kind of thing. If it was a stranger, it might be differ-ent. But someone I was involved with, it's different. I mean, if someone was trying to rob me on the street and they happened to be a woman and they struck me, I might hit back, but not someone I was involved with. I don't know why there is that difference, but that's just the way I feel.

Were your parents ever violent?

No, not physically. In my family, it was rare for anyone to even raise their voice.

What do you know about her parents?

Her natural father and mother were not violent, to my knowledge. She had two stepfathers, and they were both physically violent. Her first hus-band and her second husband were both physically violent. So, it was some-thing she was used to. It was not something I was used to.

Jake T., a construction worker, had a similar attitude toward hitting back. He is 30 years old. He was married for just three years and has one child from his marriage. He is over six feet tall, and his ex-wife is only five feet three inches. Throughout their marriage, his wife used drugs, mainly amphetamines. She worked sporadically as a waitress:

I think a lot of her problems had to do with the drug use. I mean, I could never tell when she might come unglued. It would happen all of a sudden, usually in the bedroom. For example, one night I was sitting on the side of the bed, taking off my shoes, and she just came at me, kicking and swinging, no warning, nothin'. Just bang, she starts in. That's the way it was with her. She would never say why.

One time, she did throw a knife at me, It missed, but most of the time, she would hit with her fists and kick. I'd just either hold her arms, or put up my arms, and then leave, till she had a chance to settle down. Later, if I mentioned what she did, she'd hardly ever talk about it. First, she would say she was sorry and stuff.

I did think about hitting her back, but it's just not in my nature. I just thought it would make things worse. I just knew it wouldn't be right, morally. I guess in the back of my mind, I knew it wouldn't do me any good, and that I would be worse off legally, but that's not the reason I didn't do it.

Hiding It

Jeff W.:

I guess I never really got hurt real bad. After all, I was a lot bigger than she was, and I could usually always hold her arms. Once though, she did catch me unexpectedly, and I ended up with a real shiner of an eye. I told the guys at work I had slipped on some oil, fixing my car, and banged into the bumper.

One commonality with many women victims of domestic abuse is that abused men often hide evident injuries from friends and family with other explanations. Saying they had banged into an open door when getting out of bed seemed to be a fairly frequent explanation for head bruises; scratches were explained as coming from an animal; and so forth. *Men Don't Tell* is indeed an appropriate title for a movie on the subject of abused men. According to the producer of this 1994 CBS television film, more women than men watched it.[5] In the British sample survey by Malcolm George, the overwhelming majority disguised their injuries as coming from an accident instead of from an abusive spouse. Engbritson says that there is a great similarity in the experiences between battered men and women hiding their situation from others and those who are chemically dependent:

There is denial of a problem that the person in the situation thinks they should be able to handle on their own. There is isolation because of the sense of shame that the problem is not one they can handle, but they are not prepared to seek out help because they don't know where to go to get that help, but they also don't seek out the help, until it gets to a certain point, or others insist they get help.

Engbritson says the syndrome leads to a common rationale for both battered men and women:

For the man with apparent physical injuries, they would make excuses, just as battered women often do. If someone would ask about, say, their black eye, they would say that they walked into a door or something. They will say that if they had handled it differently, or hadn't acted the way they did, then the abuse would not have happened.

One of the men I interviewed, Jason M., explained it best:

I made excuses for years, really. I'd say to myself, or even to her, "That's O.K....It was just because you had a really bad day at work, and the kids were especially cranky." Things like that. I'd talk to her about it after things had settled down, and she'd promise not to hit at me or throw things ever again, and then we'd make up. Of course, it did happen again.

Did you blame yourself for what happened?

Yeah, I would blame myself, too, you bet. After one of her blowups, I'd try to think of things that I could make right. Like one time, she threw a piece of wood at me in the garage, when she got her shoe dirty on some oil on the floor. Geez, you gotta expect that on a garage floor, you know? It wasn't like it was a big puddle or anything. But it was my job to keep the garage clean, so I made sure that there was a pad down over where the car was usually parked. But, it didn't matter. She kind of skidded in stepping on the pad. Maybe I should have used kitty litter....Whoops, you see what I mean? I'm still doing it! Anyway, she kind of skidded on the pad I guess, and she yells at me from the garage, "I thought I told you to clean this shit up, not just cover it up, you idiot!" Like that you know. I just couldn't do anything right, and I knew that when she got back that she would still be angry and any little excuse would be found, and she might throw something. I'd walk around the house on tiptoes, trying all the time to make sure things were just right, but there was no pleasing her sometimes. It was like she would just get locked into this thing, and there was nothing I could do.

Steve J. says he never told anyone about what was going on, but he had trouble explaining why not: "I don't know. I really don't know. I guess I just didn't feel comfortable about it. Maybe it was because I didn't want to admit to myself it was happening."

Would it have been embarrassing?

Yeah, that might be part of it, that I let it happen, that I didn't stand up and be a man, you know....My family, well, we have all kinds of communication problems in my family. My mom's an alcoholic, dad's kind of one of those closed, stoic, father-figure types—easy communication was not really possible in my family. My sister, who I was probably the closest to, is a gossip, and anything I told her would have gone right back to my folks. So, I didn't tell her anything. No one in my family gave me any support for this marriage, so I already had a couple of strikes against me.

Tim S. suffered slapping, hitting, and having things thrown at him. He had had only one physical injury, when he was hit in the head with a frying pan. He says he never told anyone about his abuse: "Because they would assume that I had done something to her, or that I deserved it. You know, that I had gotten into the doghouse with the little missus."

Construction worker Jake T. says he talked to two people about what was happening to him:

> I did talk to one of my coworkers about it. It made me feel better to talk about it, because he was willing to listen. He said, "You should have known it was coming, because that's the way women are." I talked to a friend, actually it was her best friend, and she was more sympathetic. They couldn't understand why she did what she did; they were surprised that she would go to such extremes. In fact, this friend said that she would have knocked her block off, and wanted to step in, and said, "Let me thump her." She really wanted to! [laughs] Other than that, I didn't tell anyone. I feel that it's a personal matter, so I don't talk about it much. There is somewhat of a fear of ridicule, because I'm afraid they might laugh at me.

Not every man hides it, however, not even the most "macho" of men, as the case of Carolina Panthers National Football League running back Fred Lane demonstrates. In the locker room, his teammates questioned him about the cuts and bruises he had. He did tell them that (his wife) Deidra did it. In 2003, she was sentenced to nearly eight years in prison for his murder. He was planning to leave her, came home to get some things, and then she shot him with a shotgun as he entered the door. As he lay dying on the floor, she shot him again.

Shame and Ridicule

No man or woman wants to admit to the world that he or she has been physically assaulted by a mate. It is just not an easy thing to do. Most people want their home to appear to the rest of the world as that of a nice, "normal" family.

For men, there is an added dimension of shame not faced by female victims. While the word *shame* was not used by any of the men I interviewed, the word that did come up time and again was *wimp*. "I didn't tell anyone because I was afraid of being called a wimp." They feared what might be said about them. Being physically abused by a woman, even though they were not supposed to hit back, was emasculating. Clearly, the victims believed that their friends, relatives, and coworkers would believe that they were not real men if they told about their abuse.

In the television movie *Men Don't Tell*, the victim sums up this feeling when he reacts to his father's puzzlement as to why he could not "control" his wife. "Are you saying I'm less of a man because a woman hits me, because I don't hit her back?"

The fear of this type of reaction is what nearly all of the victims I interviewed expressed. Mark K., who we previously heard from, suffered hitting, kicking, scratching, and being attacked with a knife. He said he only told members of his family and one friend about what was happening. He said fear of embarrassment kept him from telling other people he was close to: "Well, you know, just from being in a dysfunctional family. You don't want people to think things are wrong, bad."

Is it kind of a shameful thing?

Kind of, yeah…

Were you also embarrassed because she's a woman doing this and you're a man?

[Chuckles] Yeah, kind of…I guess it is a respect kind of thing; I was afraid I would lose respect from my friends, if I told them, for staying with someone like that. I mean, I'm a man and she's my wife, and I couldn't do anything about it. She was also stepping out on me. She made a play for my sister's boyfriend while we were still together, and I knew about that. My life-long friend, who would never lie about this kind of thing, told me after we broke up that she had made a play for him. I just didn't want people to know that I had married an outraged, alcoholic nut.

Mark K.'s chuckle before he answered the question is significant. Malcolm George, a physiologist at Queen Mary and Westfield College in England, closely examined a number of male spouse abuse victims. He noted that the victims themselves often react with laughter or humor when telling their stories:

That is protective humor. Perpetrators will point to this reaction, among male victims, and say it shows that it is no big deal, that it is obviously not a traumatic thing. But, how do they know? The humor might just be used as self-protection. The awful truth of it is so dangerous to him that he dares not admit it for his own well-being, his own self-esteem. They cannot treat it in any other way.

The conditioning of society expects men to be strong, and to show vulnerability in being attacked by a woman who supposedly is not strong enough to hurt them is something that is difficult for men to admit to. In all of the victims I have dealt with, this is a common reaction. When I first began the survey, I would get a call, and the man said he would be willing to volunteer for the survey, and I'd say, "So, you're a battered husband, are you?" Bang, the phone would go down. Or they would say, "Oh no, I'm not a victim, I'm not a victim." But then, they would go on to describe tons of times when they had been attacked. But they would firmly deny being a victim of marital violence or a battered husband. So, I began to take a different approach. I don't use the term *battered husband* if I can help it. Because *battered wife* is in the popular vernacular, the term *battered husband* has a connotation with *battered wife,* and men are put off by it. I use the term *a victim of marital violence.* It's a little more neutral.

We are conditioned in some measure by the society in which we live. In television shows, for instance, when a woman makes a deprecating or demeaning remark about a man, the audience can often be relied on to laugh. Sometimes when a woman slaps a man, applause is the result. Should a man do the same types of things, however, the reaction is usually much different. One need only watch situation comedies and even television commercials to verify this. To give but one example among many (American Furniture Warehouse, Budget Rent-A-Car, and others), an ad for Dish Network showed a man and his wife at a swimming pool. The man reads the newspaper while a woman in a bikini bends over in front of him. The man doesn't see this, and says "Wow," presumably due to a Dish Network ad in the paper. The wife, thinking he's referring to the woman in the bikini, strikes him in the jaw. If the situation was reversed and she presumably said "Wow" to the sight of an attractive male, it is doubtful the company would run an ad of him hitting her in the jaw.

Male domestic violence victims are aware of this. It has become a part of our culture; for instance, a 1963 study of 20 consecutive editions of comic strips during a month in 1950 found that husbands were the victims of hostility and attack in 63 percent of all conflict situations, while wives were victims in 39 percent.[6] It is regretful that there is apparently not a more recent examination of the comic strips in this regard, but it is doubtful that a great deal has changed. It seems, at least, that male victimization is still thought of as being funny. Although, as we shall see later in the book, that is beginning to change.

Patricia Overberg was the executive director of the Valley Oasis Emergency Shelter Program in Lancaster, California. A the time of this book's first edition, Valley Oasis was the only shelter for domestic violence in the United States that provided shelter and services for both men and women. This program is discussed in further detail in Chapter 5.

It is instructive to note what she has to say about the reactions she gets when she helps male victims or when she talks about them to groups, as she explained an interview with the author in 1996:

> One of the things that men have to deal with, that women don't have to, is indeed ridicule. I can tell you that from experience, both from working with these men, and from making speaking engagements. When I mention that we are a shelter that provides shelter to battered men, they all laugh, the men and the women. They think it's funny that a man would be battered. They laugh when I tell them that a man can be raped. Of course, I don't think it's funny at all.... I know that there are a lot of battered men out there, but part of the reason they don't seek help is this fear of ridicule.... [It] is indeed a big factor. I worked with a man who was an ironworker. Now, an ironworker is

the epitome of macho. This guy was big, and his wife was tall, but thin, probably no more than a hundred pounds. She kept putting him in the hospital. She kept beating him up with a baseball bat. Every time he came out of the hospital, they [his coworkers] were laughing him off the girders. They had no sympathy or empathy for him.

Sylvia Ashton is the chief inspector of a domestic violence police unit in England. In the news media, she has encouraged people to realize and acknowledge the fact that domestic violence does have many male victims. She relates one story of a man who was stabbed by his wife, then stabbed again because he had bled on the carpet! She says that when she tells this story to groups, the reaction is laughter.

George says Ashton's experience is not unique. He says the best way to deal with a humorous reaction is to turn the story around: "We need to say to them, 'Think of that story the other way around.' Think what you would say if I told you that there was a woman who was stabbed by her husband, and then stabbed again because she bled on the carpet. You'd say, 'What an awful bastard that man is, and I hope he went away for life,' etc."

Controlling Behavior

George says that while the ridicule male victims often experience is more intense and of a different type from what female victims experience, controlling behavior is an area that seems quite similar. Two-thirds of those he interviewed were clearly in a relationship where the physical abuse was a means to establish control:

They might not have used the word *control,* but they certainly identified such behavior, bullying, etc., as the reason behind their wife's violence. One man said that his wife used to say to him all the time, "Let me control your life." Yet, the victim very rarely recognized or would admit that what their wife was doing was controlling them, despite all the evidence. The similarities with the experiences of battered women are very strong.

A common kind of controlling behavior, according to George, is related to finances. The women often controlled the purse strings totally. It did not matter whether or not the man had the higher income. The woman made all the financial decisions, and any money given to the man, for his use, had to be justified.

Steve J., one of the men I interviewed, did mention early on that he thought his wife was very controlling:

She made all the decisions, about everything. She would decide how and where to spend money, what discipline there would be for the children, when we would make love, just everything. After a while, I began to view my own opinions as wrong. I became convinced my view was wrong all the time, so I stopped trying. Why bother, was my attitude. It just got that way after so many years. She would constantly contradict me, especially in front of the children. One thing I especially thought was bad, and I would try to talk to her about it later, although it never did any good, was about the children. I would make a decision, say about not having any TV because homework wasn't done, that kind of thing, and she would find out about it, and then overturn it, saying they could have TV. This happened constantly, and it became another area where I just gave up trying.

Tom W. is 50 years old. He was married for 15 years and has three children. He was a teacher during his marriage, but after his divorce, he left teaching and now works three jobs. He had been divorced for five years when I spoke with him. The physical abuse he suffered consisted of his wife hitting him, usually with her fists, "about once a week," usually on the shoulder or back. A knife and a hammer were also thrown at him, but throwing things was not her usual pattern. The hitting did not begin until after they had been married for 10 years:

Why did the hitting begin after you had been married for 10 years?

I don't know. I don't feel like it was anything that provoked it. I don't feel as though I am a violent person. If anything, I treated everything...probably very docile, hoping that things would improve. In retrospect, if I had been more of an authoritarian-type person, this is the type of thing she would need. She could not, or would not, make decisions, and yet the decisions I made would always be the wrong ones.

In what ways were the things you did always the wrong things?

She had a rotten habit of putting everything in the refrigerator and forgetting about it. If anybody else would come along and clean out the refrigerator, it would create a violent situation. No one could do the dishes well enough for her, and yet she wouldn't do the dishes. If I took the garbage out, I had to make sure that I at least got it off the premises. Otherwise, she would go out and get the garbage and bring it back in, with the idea that she was going to sort through it. But she never really got around to sort through it. So, it would stink. I would make it a practice of not only taking the garbage out, but I made arrangements with a neighbor to take the garbage there so it would be off the premises. She would put dirty diapers in the bathtub and leave them there, sometimes for a week. I would have to sneak in and get them out. She would make a lot of long-distance phone calls, up to four hundred dollars a month. I would question her about this, explain how we couldn't afford it, but she just ignored me. My birthday present each year was the opportunity to have sex; otherwise, it was completely refused. I gave up trying really, but if I even showed some sort of interest, or she thought I was showing an interest, this was an excuse to have an argument.

Did she work outside of the home?

No. I had suggested that she find work. But that caused quite a few problems. She accused me of just trying to get her out of the house and out of my life. I told her that wasn't the idea, that she had a good mind, and I felt as though she would be much more content. I said, "Obviously you are not happy with cooking, and doing the housework and all, but anytime I do it, it's not good enough for you. So I feel as though you'd be happier." But no, she rejected that.

With the dirty dishes situation, or other things, how did you try to work things out?

Generally, I would try to get her to sit down at the table where we could talk things out. She would start banging on the table. I would just sort of sit there passively and say, "Well, as soon as you get done, then we can go on." She would say, "Well, I'm not being unreasonable." I'd ask her to come up with some solutions, and she'd say, "I don't know. It's up to you to come up with the solutions." I'd then come up with some to try, and she'd say, "Nope, I won't do that."

If you could finally get her to tell you what she did want, and you did it the way she wanted it done, how did she react then?

She would watch me do something, and then she would go back behind me and arrange it the way it was before. If it was straightening up a room, rather than her getting in and helping, she would stand and watch. Once I had gotten books and things straightened up, she would come back and mess them up in her way rather than make them look orderly. She enjoyed it, I guess, the clutter. I received the satisfaction of at least getting the dust, and the food, that had accumulated out of there.

David L. is 41 years old. He has a daughter who was four years old when he separated from his wife. He was married for five years. He works as a freelance graphic artist, but before his separation, he worked for large corporations. His wife hit him hard enough to knock the breath out of him on one occasion, but most of the physical abuse did not involve hitting:

There was not a pattern of her beating on me. Most of the abuse in our relationship was emotional. It got more intense after the baby was born. She did hit me several times. I never responded physically, because I'm the man, and I'm supposed to be stronger than this. She slammed doors a lot. She would get into screaming fits and throw things around, but not necessarily at me. She was extremely jealous. She would physically step between me and any woman friends.

Did she say you were sexually inadequate?

Yes, usually to a third party. She would allude to that, and I would find out about her remarks later. She was a real tease to other men. She would even do that in front of me. She was really weird. One week she was crying, and she didn't feel she was attractive to men any more. She needed to prove to herself that she was. That Saturday she got dressed up more or less like a hooker and went out and cruised the malls. She said she ended up at the airport with three guys from [another state], who invited her to fly with them to [a ski resort two states away]. We were seeing this marriage counselor at this time, and he seemed to think that she needed to prove that to herself, so I let it go. But that gives you some idea of the extent to which I was willing to try to keep things on an even keel. I felt that my daughter should be able to call on either parent at any time and have us there. I learned later that she had been having an affair during the last year of our marriage, but I didn't know that at the time.

How did you respond when there was this screaming and throwing things around going on? What did you do to calm things down?

I would tell her to calm down and talk to me, but she wouldn't. She would say the outburst was not directed at me, even though it obviously was, that she was just "venting." She would imagine things. Things that she said I did but were things that I guess that her father or brothers had done. We did go to counseling for a long time, but that turned into another form of abuse. She kept demanding compromises, and I was willing to make them, but she wasn't. Every time she got a compromise from me, she would back off and say it wasn't enough. The counselor finally caught on to her manipulation. It was a way for her to gain ground without giving any.

Did the counselor ever ask you about being physically hit or abused?

No, he never did.

Did you tell him?

I don't think so.

Tell me more about any controlling behavior. In what ways was she controlling?

She was very controlling. She was extremely rigid. She decided how money was to be spent, where we'd go, who we'd see, who our friends should be. I couldn't do anything right; it didn't matter what it was. I even sent her a dozen long-stem roses one day, and she knocked that effort, too. I tried to make friends with her brother, took him out and stuff, because I could see that was important to her, but he still wouldn't speak to me. That was of course my fault, not his. I worked my butt off to try and keep her satisfied. No matter what I did, doing the dishes, cleaning, child care, it was wrong. It was a codependent relationship, I guess, and I was enabling. She took everything that I could give and threw it back in my face....It was very painful. It was far more painful than the physical abuse. I could handle myself there; it just added to the overall sense of things, kept things on edge, because I never knew for sure when it might escalate into that, too.

Did she seem to present herself one way in public and another way at home?

Yes, there was that. She was able to fool people, but at home it was a different story.

David L. mentions domestic abuse involving two aspects of controlling behavior that a number of the men commented on. They frequently remarked about the difference between public and private personas and the intentional setting up of situations by the women to see how they would react to their flirting with other men.

The Mask

Construction worker Jake T. sums up this phenomenon: "In front of others, our friends and so on, she was giggling and happy, small and dainty, but the mask came off behind closed doors."

College student Tim S. went into more detail about this aspect of his situation:

She would change all the time. You couldn't tell how she was going to react; she was very unpredictable. If we had a disagreement in public, she would not say it, not contradict me, you know, but she would hold it inside until we got home. There was this Pollyanna thing, sweet in public, but once we got home, it was a different deal. I was her first real boyfriend, she said, so she was really clingy. I guess you could say she was dependent on me physically and emotionally. Like one time, I came home to find her sitting real close to a male friend of mine, with her hand on his knee. Later he told me that he was glad when I walked in, because she was making him uncomfortable, if you know what I mean. She would do things like that. She seemed to come on to my friends, make sexual comments to them. If I complained, she'd say things like, "I'm not your property." I'd say, "No shit, but I thought we had a commitment to each other." I hate to sound Freudian, but I think she disliked or maybe hated her father, and since I was her first real boyfriend, or guy she lived with, I think she took it out on me as a male.

Because the male victim knows that many people have difficulty believing that a woman can be dangerously violent in the home, the contrast between how she might appear in public adds to their dilemma. George found that disbelief was the most common reaction of the men he interviewed. "They couldn't believe it was happening to them."

Not knowing there are other men in the same situation adds to the sense of disbelief over the contrast between the public perception of themselves and their mates as well as to the sense of isolation.

George, in an interview with the author, reported a bizarre twist to the public and private lives of victims and perpetrators. Many men were abused because their public image was not macho enough to suit the batterer:

So, the fact that the man didn't beat someone up outside of the home was reason enough to beat them up inside the home. That fact that the husband wouldn't force and bully doctors, trades people, etc., someone the couple came in contact with, was a reason for a beating. The fact that the wife wanted something done, and that it wasn't just not done, but not done in a macho enough way, meant that he was in trouble.

THE DIFFICULTY OF LEAVING

Fear of ridicule, shame, and a desire to keep family matters private prohibit many men and women from revealing their domestic abuse to others. These isolation factors also play a role in preventing the victim from leaving the abusive situation.

Responsibility

Patricia Overberg contends from her many years of experience working with both female and male victims that men not only have a more difficult time admitting they are victims and seeking help, but they also have a more difficult time leaving the abusive relationship:

It's more difficult for a man than a woman to seek help. Men have been brought up with this macho upbringing, which I think is really a great disservice to men. They have this feeling that they must protect the women. If this means that they have to take whatever the women dish out to them, they will. They'll stay. I find it very sad. They will come to our outreach group, and it takes a lot to convince them they should leave the relationship, and they should do the same things for themselves that the female victim does. It is much more difficult to get a man to make that change. They have been brought up to see their role as being defined as protector of the home. When you get married it's your responsibility to provide, to make sure there is food on the table, clothes. Regardless of the fact that women are going out and working these days, men are still taught that it is their responsibility to provide. So, if you leave, you are abdicating your responsibility, and you are less than a man (interview with the author).

Mark K. says this sense of responsibility was the primary reason he didn't leave his marriage sooner:

I just didn't want to see the breakup. I know that the whole root of her problem is her alcoholism, and I was always hoping it would stop and change. I did get her to stop for a while. I think that's what brought on a lot of the fights, and because I tried to stop it, she ended up sneaking around and stuff. I loved the woman. Even after everything that has happened, I still love her, and I don't know how to change that.

Did you feel responsible, as a man, for the family?

Yes, definitely. Just like when she quit working. I said to heck with it, stay home, take care of the baby—I'll just work overtime; and that's what I did.

Did you blame yourself?

For not being there a lot of times, yeah, I did. I worked twelve to fourteen hours a day sometimes, six days a week.

Curt Engbritson, in an interview with the author, says this sense of responsibility to the family unit, in the traditional role of male provider, provides a major roadblock to leaving the relationship:

One man was not even married to this abusive spouse, but he stayed out of a sense of obligation to the children, who were not his biological children. He felt fearful for his life, because she had a gun and had threatened him with it. Still, he stayed because he felt it was his responsibility to help care for the children. He finally did leave.

This sense of responsibility prevents many from leaving. They do keep thinking that it will get better, so they stay on. One man left the relationship, but the woman convinced him that she had changed, so he returned. She became pregnant and gave birth to twins. He is still in that relationship, which has never ceased to be abusive. His sense of obligation to the family prevented him from leaving initially, then when he did go back, his obligations increased.

Codependency, guilt, a pattern of learned behaviors from the relationship, and their own family enforces the sense of responsibility that these men have.

Children

For the male victims with children, leaving an abusive relationship becomes especially difficult. They strongly believe that it is their responsibility to provide for the children, and in many cases, they acted as protector of the children when their spouse was abusive to them as well.

They also strongly believe that the judicial system is stacked against them because of their gender and that gaining custody of the children will be difficult if not impossible. Many believe that physical custody will be won by their spouse and that any visitation granted will be blocked or denied by their spouse in a continuation of controlling and abusive behavior. They also fear that the "atom bomb" of child custody disputes might be dropped on them: being accused of sexually molesting their child. Unfortunately, the circumstances of several men interviewed bear out these beliefs.

The first interview in this section involves a number of issues besides those concerned with children and is told in greater length than most of the other interviews presented; however, most of the issues in this case do revolve around the children. Also, I want to present at least one interview in this chapter "in total" so as to give the full flavor of a long chain of events.

James J. is 40 years old and was married to Betty in 1981. They had two children. They lived in a suburb of a large city in a western state. They are currently divorced. She had a six-figure income as a physician (her actual profession), and he was a homemaker while the children were small. They agreed that since her income was higher and he could use the computer at home for much of his work, this was a good arrangement. When the children got older, the agreement was that she would help support his further higher education. She controlled all spending decisions.

During the first years of marriage, she would sometimes block him from leaving a room. He would sometimes push his way past her, but that is as aggressive as he became in response. "I didn't recognize at the time that was symptomatic of being violent and controlling," James says. Both became involved in women's issues at their church, involving women as ministers and using gender-neutral language. During one episode, he was writing a suggested revision for such language on the computer. They had a disagreement over how to phrase things, and she grabbed his hair and pulled his neck and back sharply over the chair. He was sore for several days.

Another time, she decided to bake a cake for their three-year-old son's birthday. She couldn't find a particular pan, and she began screaming at James for not knowing exactly where it was. She began cursing and hitting him in the stomach and chest. He raised his arms to ward off the blows. His mother was present during this scene. He grabbed his son to take him away from the cursing. Betty blocked their way, but he left the kitchen through a side door. She picked up a heavy padlock and threw it at him while he had the child in his arms. It missed. Later, his son asked him, "Why does mommy hit you?"

She constantly belittled his role as a homemaker and would often scream, yell, curse, and hit him. He never struck back. She would often take the car keys so he could not leave the house. James says, "I later learned from talking to domestic violence counselors that taking keys is a control thing that is really typical of abusers." He began to experience stress-related health problems. He asked her to attend marriage counseling with him, but she refused and would become angry when he even brought up the subject.

The police were called after several altercations, but they never arrested her; they simply took a report and left. After eight years of marriage, she filed for divorce. The children were five and three years old. He stayed in the house while the divorce was pending, and she left the children with him. He received no funds from her except for $2,000 he was able to withdraw from an automatic teller machine. James says:

> My attorney was no use. She was slow to act and never requested a restraining order against her. There was an initial agreement between attorneys that both sides were not to remove the children from the home without mutual agreement, and no property was to be removed. However, she violated this anyway and took a whole bunch of property and nearly all the children's clothes. I was keeping the children most of the time, so this was very hard.

He went to her workplace to videotape the clothes and other property that he knew she had in her car; he wanted to prove she was violating the court-approved agreement. She came out and saw him doing this. He buckled the seat belt in the driver's seat to prevent her from removing him from the car, which was at that point still legally half his. She pushed him face down over on the passenger side of the front seat, while he was still buckled in, and got on top of his back. She kicked his lower back with her knees, scratched his face, tried to get the keys out of his pocket, and began yelling to a coworker in the parking lot that he was stealing the car and to call the police. He had a cellular phone with him and tried to call his attorney so that when the police arrived, the attorney could tell them that he co-owned the car. She grabbed his phone and beat him over the head with it. When the police came, they refused to take a report, even though he had blood streaming down his face and was in obvious pain. James says, "If it had been a man beating up a woman, they would have made an arrest. They said, 'We ain't taking no report from you buddy.'" The police told him to get out of there or be arrested for car theft, despite the fact that he did show them papers that named him as coinsurer of the car.

He went to the hospital emergency room, where his most apparent wounds were treated. Later, he saw a doctor and found that one rib was fractured and several ribs were bruised and out of alignment. He also had a groin injury, many bruises, and muscle injuries. James says:

I had read in *M.S.* magazine that if you are the victim of a domestic assault, you should get treatment, take photographs, which I had a friend do, and call a domestic violence shelter. So I spent several hours that evening calling, saying, "This is what happened. The police refuse to take a report. I need a restraining order. How can I get her arrested?" They said, "Well, we don't know what to say to a man." Or, "Well, we just help women." I wasn't asking to be checked into one of their shelters—that's another issue; I was just asking for advice on how to deal with this procedurally, with the police and courts and so on. I asked, "Well, what would you say to a woman in this situation?" They would refuse to answer my questions because I am male. I learned later that domestic violence shelter workers are trained to take calls from men as crank calls. From their perspective, if a man calls, claiming to be a victim, it's actually a perpetrator trying to get information on how to beat the system. It raises a lot of significant questions about agencies that receive government funding yet discriminate on the basis of sex.

Finally I called a sexual assault crisis line and talked to a wonderful counselor. I told her that this wasn't a sexual assault but asked if she could help. She said she recognized that men, too, can be victims of domestic violence, and she told me exactly what to do—which numbers to call at the police department and what to ask for, with very detailed instructions. She said if that doesn't work, she would call on my behalf. She was calming and very supportive. I did what she told me, and within an hour the police came and took a report.

The police told me that they could call and get an emergency restraining order right then, but they talked me out of it. They said I didn't really need it, that I could wait the weekend, until court opened on Monday. They assured me that since they had taken a report, I could call the watch commander and my wife could be arrested if she came near me. I was more fortunate than many domestic violence victims, as I was able to be in a secure building with my parents and the children were with me. My wife came to the building several times, demanding to be let in, but we refused.

It was still very hard, as it was a one-bedroom apartment and very cramped with two small children and my parents and me.

On Sunday, I went home with the children but barricaded the doors, just like in the movies. She came to the door with a male friend, whom I didn't know, and began pounding on the door, opening it with her key and demanding to be let in. I did what the police told me to do. I called the watch commander and gave him the report number, expecting they would come out and arrest her. Did they arrest her? No, they insisted that I let her in.

They called another officer, who was the very same one who refused to take a report at the parking lot beating. It was obvious they were buying everything she told them. The police did let me and the kids stay in the house, and they told her to stay elsewhere, after making sure she had a place to stay.

The only thing that worked in my favor was that the police found me in the house initially, and it was obvious from talking to the kids that I was the primary caretaker. Otherwise, I'm sure I would have been the one kicked out of the house and probably arrested, too.

The attack happened on Friday; Sunday I went to the house and had the scene with her and the police. On Monday, I tried to get in touch with my attorney, but she never got back to me, and I told her receptionist that she was fired. After getting the kids settled at a friend's house, because I was afraid she would kidnap them if I took them to their regular preschool or left them at home, I spent hours at the courthouse. I kept getting the bureaucratic runaround there but made it to the right place to get a restraining order after filling out the paperwork. Then I was told I couldn't get one because I had an attorney of record and couldn't file on my own. I told them I had fired that attorney, but that was no good because I hadn't filled out the proper paperwork to fire the attorney. I was almost in tears. I ran into a woman in the hall who was going through the same kinds of problems, and we sort of commiserated with each other. Part of my point is that the system is bad for victims of domestic violence, but it is worse for men. At least there are some resources available for women, although it's not easy or good for them either.

I went home, and my son began asking questions about why he couldn't go to school and why we were staying at this house, and so on. I had told him Friday that it was a stranger who had beaten me up. This time, I decided to tell him the truth. I said, "You know, I told you it was a stranger who beat me up. It wasn't; it was mommy. The reason why you're here is because I'm trying to go to court to have the judge say that mommy can't take you away and that she can't hit me or take things from home, and that's why you're here, and that's why you're not going to school." I decided, after that, that I would always tell my children the truth. That there were some things I might shelter them from if I could, but if they were aware of it, and asking about it, I would not lie to them. I didn't want to lose my integrity, and their confidence in me, on top of everything else I was losing.

On Tuesday, I finally got into court to seek a restraining order. I took in the documentation of the injuries from the doctor and the emergency room, the pictures of the injuries, and the judge also had copies of the police report. She [Betty] and my new attorney met with the judge in chambers. My attorney came out and told me the judge looked at the pictures, laughed, and said, "Well, you have to expect one knock-down drag-out fight per divorce; let's keep these two apart." Betty had made no allegations of my having attacked her, yet the judge took a neutral stance of "We can't tell who hit who" and made the restraining order mutual. My attorney told me, "Don't bring up this thing about you being a victim of domestic violence again. The judge will view you as a wimp, and you'll lose custody of the kids." I said, "What you're telling me is that she could beat me to a bloody pulp, leave me disabled so I couldn't care for the kids, and she could get custody because I couldn't care for them?" He said, "That's about right; that's the way it goes."

The judge ordered that I would be in the house for a week, and she would be in for a week, and the children would stay there, with de facto joint custody. Neither one of us was supposed to remove any property from the house except personal clothing and toiletries. I later learned that, under the law, the police were supposed to have arrested her, on the spot, since she was the non-injured party. Had she not been a woman, I am sure the result in court would have been much different as well. A man would have been restrained and prevented from entering the house; would have received very limited visitation, if any; and would have been ordered to immediately pay support, both spousal support and child support. I did get a small amount of spousal support, which was unusual for a man, but it was about half the usual amount a woman would have gotten, given Betty's income. The only thing I got, besides that, was that she had to rent me a car until she gave me enough money to buy one, but she got the family car.

By agreement, I had taken the children on a trip to visit relatives for a week. When I got back, the house had been stripped. There was no silverware, towels were gone, all the furniture, photographs, tools, the TV and stereo, even family heirlooms of mine. You know, our garage had been burglarized once before, and there is a sense of violation when that happens, but when it is done by someone you know, there is an even greater sense of violation. Even though I was dirt poor, I spent several hundred dollars on basic kitchen stuff so I could cook for myself and the children, but stuff would continually disappear. Every week, after she got in there, stuff would go. The children's car seats, their clothes, everything would just disappear.

I repeatedly asked my attorney to get her cited for contempt, but I had these wimps for attorneys, and nothing was ever done about it. They always put me off. I later learned that under the state law a victim of domestic violence can even leave the state for their own protection, regardless of any custody order, and just inform the district attorney of their whereabouts. I also learned later that domestic violence can be a significant factor in awarding of custody. I didn't know any of that at the time; my attorney never told me or talked about this. I later learned that most of my attorney's clients were upper-middle-class females.

We had almost an entire year of this week-in, week-out hell with things disappearing from the house. The marital status was finished in a couple of months, but custody, support, and property issues took nearly a year to settle. All the ending of the marriage did was allow me to go out and marry someone else, which, of course, I was far from ready to do, and it meant I no longer had health insurance.

About six months later we had a hearing on property issues and spousal support. The judge asked me about my career plans. I told him that I was working on building up a consulting practice in my home (which I had experience in), using the computer, fax, and modem, so I could be at home most of the time to take care of the kids.

The judge (who is in his seventies), looks at me and says, "'Young man, you need to go out and get a regular job, and fulfill a more traditional father role. Your children will respect you more, and you'll be living nearby and you'll have continuing and frequent contact." My attorney says, "Your honor, this is the family law of the 1990s. There's no husband, there's no wife, it's a spouse; it's supposed to be neutral." And the judge responds with, "I'm still having difficulty adjusting to this new social order."

I later submitted that quote, from the transcript, to the county commission for women. The staff wouldn't help me, and they admitted that their role was not to help in cases of sex discrimination but only to help women who were being discriminated against on the basis of sex by county agencies. However, I did go over the staffs' head, and one of the commissioners did write a letter of protest to the supervising judge. It had no legal effect, but it was moral support.

I also filed a complaint against the police for not taking a report after the attack in the car. At first, there was no response, and I just got a very patronizing brush-off. Later, there was a [highly publicized case of alleged police misconduct based on discrimination], and I got a call from a high-ranking police officer. I also had complained to the citizens' police review commission. They later wrote me that there would be no result from them, because the officer had already been disciplined. That's the only way I found out that there had been some action taken against that officer, but I never did find out what kind of discipline it was.

Nearly a year after the attack in the car, there was a trial on custody. I was ordered out of the house. My ex-wife was awarded sole legal and physical custody. In [this state where there is joint-custody presumption], sole legal custody is rare. I am now paying $250 a month to her for child support, though she has a six-figure income. My income is under $30,000 a year. She continually blocks my visitation, and there has had to be lots of expensive letters sent by my attorney to her attorney, getting her to live up to what the court ordered for visitation. My youngest daughter has not gained any weight in the two years since my ex-wife got custody.

Nearly two years later, she attacked me again. It was my weekend with the kids, and we were at [a public event], and my ex-wife was there, too. I just kept my distance. The kids had told me that they were going with her to put the family pet to sleep. I think that's something the kids should be told about, but I think taking the dog to the vet should be something adults should do, as it's traumatic enough. But she's very good at manipulating, so if I said no, then I would be blamed for not letting the kids say a last good-bye. Anyway, I took my four-year-old daughter over to where she was eating with my son. Even though it was my visitation time, I take the position that it's O.K., that I wouldn't prevent the children from seeing her if there was something that they wanted to do with her, as long as I got some makeup time. She told me about going to the vet with the kids, and I asked her for how long, etc., and I said O.K.—as long as I get an equivalent amount of extra time next week. Well, she went ballistic. She complained about me violating court orders and called me a "fucking asshole" in front of the kids. I'm trying to back away and she grabs my necktie. You know, there's a lot of jokes about a woman grabbing a man's tie, but I like to turn it around. Suppose it's a man grabbing a woman's long scarf around her neck as she's trying to move away? Is that going to be viewed as a joke? I don't think so. She jerked hard and prevented my getting away. I view that as a physical attack.

That was the latest. I filed a complaint about violating the court order against physical attacks and using derogatory language about one another in front of the children. She filed a counterclaim, and the judge ruled against my petition for contempt but didn't uphold her counterclaim of filing unnecessary suits.

The bottom line is she's fat and happy. I'm deeply in debt; I've never received any of the community property I'm supposed to get, and she has sole custody of the children. She's in complete denial about [one of her relative's] history of sexual abuse of children, even though I submitted a letter to the court from a child he had abused. My daughter has complained to me about him touching her, and I told her to say no, and then say "no" loudly and complain to an adult. She told me, "Daddy, I can't say no, mommy won't let me." So, there's this pattern of intimidation, control, and denial in her family, and I think that's where it's coming from. Several psychologists who have talked to her, and me, say the anger she exhibits could not possibly have come from something I've done; it comes from her and her background. I'm still going to try to change custody, but it doesn't look good.

I've moved, and I'm asking a local council on domestic violence to adopt a policy that says there shall be no discrimination in provision of services against anyone on the basis of religion, sexual orientation, race, physical handicap, or gender. I think they'll adopt it. I don't know of any state in the nation where it's legal for an agency that accepts government funds to discriminate on the basis of sex. Maybe you could argue for a separate but equal basis, though that's a very tenuous argument, too. How can a feminist, or anyone, argue for sex discrimination? Yet that's exactly what's going on in shelters and crisis lines across the country.

Tom W. was married for 15 years and has three children. His wife was emotionally and physically abusive to him, and she was emotionally abusive to the children. When asked what the "final straw" incident was that made him take action to separate, he told me the following incidents and what happened involving the children:

> Her mother came to visit, and her brother. They ended up staying quite a long time. All of a sudden, we had a house full of people. For some reason—my wife didn't have any proof—I was accused of playing around. I don't know with whom. They took it upon themselves to go before the [school board members] and accuse me of playing around with somebody. There was no evidence at all. This caused quite a bit of distress. I didn't want the [school] to be caught in the middle of this domestic matter, so it eventually led to my leaving [teaching].
>
> Her mother went back to [where she lived in another state], but her brother stayed. He went to child protection services and said I was abusing the children, sexually abusing them. I had to go to the authorities, but it was proven that in no way had I sexually abused them; if anyone had, it was this uncle, and he was just trying to do a cover-up. We did go through the divorce, and both child protective services and mental health were on her side. At that time, the littlest one was two months old, and they felt, and the judge agreed, that the baby should go with the mother and not break up the family. But there were different times during this, and afterwards, where there was abuse to the children. I made many complaints to child protective services and the juvenile department, but my reports were completely ignored. I did not have the money to go back into court, and I'm still at that point.

To change custody?

> Yes, or even to prove that the sexual abuse was coming from this uncle. That has accelerated in this last couple of months in that he has gone back into the home. My youngest daughter feels very unsafe. But there's really nothing I can do about it. My two oldest daughters are very concerned about her being in that environment. I feel as though I have nowhere to turn. I've gone to legal aid, and because they helped her at first, they can't help me. Mental health, child protective services, the social workers, all of them said we were supposed to do certain things. I always complied, but she never did. They would always accept her excuses.

I'm having trouble understanding the chain of events. You're saying that before the divorce the state mental health department and child protective services were investigating the charges against you, and they were disproved?

> Well, yes and no before court. I was accused by this uncle of sexually molesting my two oldest daughters. But it wasn't really until we got to family court on custody, when my two daughters testified that I had not done this, but it was this uncle, that I was really cleared. But this situation seemed

to go right over the top of the head of this judge. My attorney was very disappointed. Both my daughters are still, even today, very upset.

Was this uncle at least removed from the home, a restraining order put against him, or something?

Yes. I got a restraining order put against him from being in the home, but my former wife completely ignored that. It was almost as if it was like a challenge to her. She never accepted the fact that he sexually abused the children.

Couldn't anything be done when the restraining order was violated by this man, either by the district attorney or child protective services?

They would get in touch with my former wife, and she would say no, that he just stopped by for a few minutes and so forth. In reality, he was staying there two to three weeks at a time. They did not send out anyone to really visually see. When I would request this, they would always say, "We don't have enough people to cover that kind of thing," to see if he was really there.

The district attorney was not interested in prosecuting this man?

No, they didn't do anything, even after my two oldest daughters testified in court.

So the two oldest daughters are now out of the home, but the youngest, who is now fifteen, is still in the home?

Yes, and this uncle makes her very nervous and afraid. He opens the door to her room without knocking, things like that. She has, when she felt it was safe to, mentioned this type of thing to her mother, but her mother makes excuses for him.

What is your visitation like?

[My former wife] is still very controlling. She enjoys the power she has. I've been denied visitation many, many times. She had moved to [nearly seventy miles away], and I would get there, and I couldn't see the children because they had done something, or not done something that she wanted them to do. I'd try calling the police about this type of thing, but there's nothing they would do, because it's a civil domestic situation, and I was told I would have to go back to family court. Well, that still meant I would lose my weekend visitation, and going back to court meant an expense, and lawyers, and I just couldn't afford it. This would happen time and time again. Even now, my two oldest daughters have offered to pick up my youngest and bring her to visit me, but their mother will not permit that. I have to appear on the doorstep. My parents have offered to go and pick up my daughter, and she would love to visit with them, but the mother will not allow this.

My visitations are many times interrupted by something that the mother feels is more important, usually a church event. The daughter doesn't feel these things are all that necessary for her to attend, but she doesn't want to defy her mother. So, I say O.K. It certainly cramps the weekend. I don't dare tell the mother if I am going to spend time in [her area] because the mother will shadow us. If she knows that we are going to [a certain shopping mall], I can look around, and there's the mother standing there, watching us.

There's a lot of different things that keeps things on edge and stirred up.

David L. was married for five years and has a daughter who was four years old when he separated from his wife. His wife hit him several times, but he says there was not a pattern of her beating him; most of the abuse was emotional. She would scream and throw things around but not necessarily throw things at him. He said she was very controlling. The incident that he called the "final straw" was initiated by his wife and led to a series of events with the judicial and social service systems involving his daughter:

[My wife] would do incredible things, with the help of her mother and brother, who had virtually moved in with us. Before the divorce, they had a garage sale to get rid of my things. I would walk out into the yard, and they would lock the door behind me. I had to carry another set of keys. They set the diet and the time we would eat. We shifted to a foreign diet [his wife was Indonesian]. I didn't like smoking, so they would sit out on the patio to smoke when I was there, but they would smoke inside the house when I was gone. It was right after this garage sale thing that she basically just picked a fight. She yelled at me for using the wrong set of scissors to trim my finger-nails, and she just got right in my face. I tried to defuse things, but she kept going. She said she wanted to smoke, so we went out on the patio, and she blew smoke right in my face. I took her cigarette away from her, just took it out of her hand. She picked up the pack to get another one. I took that, too. I just reached around her. I did not in any way manhandle her at all. I barely touched her. She said, "Aha! That's assault." She called 911. I heard from people since this time that she had called a shelter and really fed them a line, and she was told what to do. It was entrapment. All I did was take her damn cigarettes. She got a restraining order. She told me the clerk at the court-house encouraged her to put down everything she could think of. She said the clerk actually told her that there was no penalty for lying. She put down I was a black belt in Karate. Bullshit. I took a few lessons in the sixties. She said I had a collection of knives. I had a few Swiss army knives, and a Bowie knife that she gave me. She said I was a gun nut. Well, as a hobby I shot black powder antique muzzle-loaders. I didn't even have a modern gun.

Two days later, the deputies came and put me in my car and said I couldn't go back. All I got was my shaving gear. She and her family had my house and my baby. That was the last time I had access to my house and belongings. They kept what they wanted and put what they didn't want outside for me to get. Like books, they'd just let sit in the rain. I had a lot of books, but they didn't value books.

I had thought because I had tried to live an honorable life, and do the right thing, and be a good parent, that someone would look at that and consider it. But no one even looked at that. I was just out.

Was there a hearing on the restraining order?

No, there wasn't. My attorney said we could go for one, but the judge certainly wouldn't throw her and the baby out. The judge would say that there might not be any basis for the restraining order as stated, but there are obvious severe problems in the relationship, and that there was no reason for me to go back into the house. That would have been another $500 to $1,000 to have a useless hearing, so I didn't see any point in it, based on what my attorney said.

What happened next?

I went to New York on a job assignment. When I got back, there were divorce papers waiting for me. My lawyer's legal assistant, who's a really savvy, salty gal, pulled me aside early on and told me: "You might as well get ready for it. At some point she's going to charge you with sexual abuse of your daughter." I said, "She's crazy, but she's not that crazy." Well, the legal assistant knew better than I did.

Where did you live after you were forced out of your home?

I stayed with my brother for about three months, then got an apartment.

How long after the restraining order was filed before you were accused of sexual abuse? How was the case made?

In [about six months later], I had my daughter for a visitation. She was still in diapers. I noticed her having trouble; she was grunting hard, and I asked her *if* she had to go poop. She said she didn't, but later I did change her diaper, and it was obvious that she was really constipated. It was a really hard but large stool. I took her home.

Two days later I got a call from my lawyer saying that I had been charged. The lawyer couldn't tell me much about it except that she had been examined by a doctor, and that it had gone to child protective services. I was totally in shock. The lawyer told me not to talk to anyone about it. Well, I had to tell the people at school and the dean [he was teaching several courses in his field]; I didn't want them to hear about it through rumors and gossip.

I knew that if my daughter had been molested that I hadn't done it, so therefore she was not being protected from whoever had done it. I thought it might be the brother, or the day care, I didn't know. I was really worried. It just drove me crazy. I would absolutely step in front of a bullet for that little girl, but nobody would tell me anything.

Finally, I called the doctor. I had at least met the doctor. She said that [the daughter's] anus had seemed a little bit swollen and distended when she examined her. That could be from molestation. I told her about her being constipated and passing a very large, hard stool, and she said that could do it, too.

I called up [my wife] and asked her about it and asked why she didn't ask me about it. Well, apparently it was just too convenient for her. She had still been going to [a local women's shelter]. I guess she liked the sympathy she got, and someone must have told her that this was a way to get custody. Who knows what she said. I do know that [the shelter] called my lawyer, who is a very well-known feminist lawyer, and chewed her out for defending me.

Next, my daughter starts going to this psychologist who became convinced that my daughter was molested. She never called me, or wanted to talk to me, until I called and insisted that I meet with her. I was looking at three to five years hard time. My lawyer got me set up right away with a lie detector test. I think that was to prove to herself, more than anything else, that I was innocent.

Then I went to see [another psychologist]. I took all these tests. I was hooked up to the peter-meter—the plethysmograph it's called and forced to look at all these dirty pictures, to see if I got an erection. You had to listen to audio fantasies on headphones. I passed that test.

How did it make you feel, going through that?

I'm still affected by it. I've talked to several other clinical psychologists since, and they don't think this test, the plethysmograph, peter-meter, has any validity. That is, it won't really tell whether anyone is a molester or not, guilt or innocence. It has left me virtually impotent. I have a relationship now with a wonderful woman, but I am just…, but every time I think about sex…I think, oh no! I mean that test…I can't even enter into a therapeutic relationship with a psychologist anymore, because of what those jerks did to me. I think [the psychologist who did the testing] is just collecting his own dirty little secrets on people. I think it's just his own highly sophisticated and extremely expensive voyeurism. It was incredibly violating. I think it's the modern-day equivalent of the old trial by fire.

So, you passed the test anyway.… There must have been a custody evaluation—was there? Did a psychologist interview both sides?

Yes, and she was excellent…a saint. She saw right through things. She said my wife was manifestly unstable and that I would provide the better upbringing for my child. There was another psychologist's report that said my wife was borderline narcissistic, had high psychomotor activity, and some other things. They brought in another psychologist who had never talked to me and attempted to characterize me. But since he had not seen both sides, I think his testimony didn't count for much.

All this was brought out in court?

Yes. I won custody. She was even chewed out by the judge. The judge asked her, "Why did you charge this man with abusing your child? Why did you deny visitation? Why did you do it? Did you really think he had done something?" My ex just stood there and said, "Well, I hoped he hadn't." Well, she obviously hoped to make other people believe I had.

What were the other parts of the ruling?

My ex got the house. She sold it to a friend for way under what it was worth. I got a few thousand for my share after paying off the lawyers and the psychologists.

How long did all this take? From the time you were charged to the judge's final ruling?

It took…, a year and a half. But it wasn't over.

It wasn't over?

No, the psychologist appointed by the court to oversee the transition from my ex having custody to me having custody required supervised visitation only. This was after my daughter told her, and everyone, "My daddy didn't do anything, but my mommy told me he did."

So you could only have supervised visitation, even after you had been given complete custody?

Right, since [this psychologist] had been my daughter's counselor, she was to supervise the change in custody, and she thought this should be a gradual change. Which I can understand, but not supervised visitation only—after I had been proven innocent.

How long did this go on?

I was only allowed a one-hour visit for a couple of weeks in her waiting room. Then I was allowed to go with a friend, who she had agreed was acceptable and who my daughter knew, to go out for ice cream…for an hour, once a week. That was allowed for a couple more weeks. Then I was allowed one overnight visit a week for a couple more weeks. During one of these stays, my daughter had a pretty severe nose bleed. I became so concerned that I took her to the hospital. I called the day care lady to see what had happened, if anything, that day, and she told me that my daughter had had a nose bleed spontaneously after getting up from her nap. Well, my daughter told me it was because she and the day care lady's son had bumped heads, and her nose got hit. I didn't trust this lady who was taking care of her, but it was someone my wife had chosen, so there was nothing I could do about it right then.

I mention this because it shouldn't have been as traumatic a thing as it was. I mean, I took her to the hospital, but I could just see those bastards saying, "He hit her in the nose." This was the type of thing I was going through. This stuff has repercussions far beyond what goes on in court and between the lawyers. You should not have to be a parent and wonder how child protective services is going to take a child's bloody nose, unless you've been a bad parent.

So you had one-hour supervised visitation for a month, then one overnight stay a week for another month. What happened next?

Well, my wife announces that she is going to move away to [a large city in an adjacent state, about 800 miles away]. So there was going to be no place else for my daughter to stay. At about this same time, to my extreme relief, I found out that [the child's psychologist] was not covered under my insurance. Under the recommendation of the psychologist who did the custody evaluation, another counselor was recommended to this psychologist, which she approved of, and this new person was placed in charge of the transition thing.

What did the new psychologist recommend?

She saw right through things. She's a saint in my book. She saw no reason to keep this artificial separation going on and allowed my daughter to move in with me right away, and anyhow my ex was moving out of town, which she did about three weeks later. She was ordered to pay $400 a month in child support for four months, then it was to increase to $518 a month. She made one payment of $400 and then stopped. Her paycheck was garnished, so one partial payment was made, then she quit the job. That was it. As we speak, she's more than $10,000 in arrears.

I have been going through hoops like you wouldn't believe to try to get any kind of enforcement of it. I finally contacted the support enforcement division supervisor in [the state where she lives], and they sent me a letter saying action would be taken. [Note: After this interview, Mark called me to say that an indictment and warrant were issued for his ex on criminal failure to pay child support; it took a year for this action to occur.]

Has there been visitation?

Yeah, she flies up here for visits and takes her back. Like during Easter vacation, she did all this flying on short-term tickets, not advance tickets, but says she can't afford to pay child support. Financially, this has been devastating. I'm a single parent, which really cuts into my ability to work. For a year there, I was really limited as my work does involve a lot of short-term traveling. Until I got my present girlfriend, I was really stuck. She and my daughter get along really great; she's a school counselor, and they really like each other. I'm now able to leave my daughter with her for short assignments out of town, which allows me to work, but it was especially difficult, with all the debts for lawyers, losing my home, and so on.... Meanwhile, child protective services still thinks I'm a child molester.

Tell me about that. I thought it was settled.

No. Like I said, the shelter where my wife had gone and fed them a lot of bull called my lawyer after it was all over and raked her over the coals for defending me. Well, apparently, the shelter and the lady assigned to the case for child protective services have been talking and supporting each other's views. I have friends who know this lady—she's a man-hater. I have tried to talk to her, get any records they have changed, close the case in other words, but I've gotten nowhere. Somewhere there are still these records that I am a suspected child molester. I told my lawyer and she called, but this lady doesn't want to hear about it. She's convinced without ever having spoken to me that I must be this horrible person. She told my lawyer that I must be a monster. That was the term my lawyer told me she used.

As far as I can tell, it's still an open case with them, so I'm still looking over my shoulder, afraid of the parent police, who can take my daughter away from me on their whim. I think that what actually happened was that my ex fantasized the possibility of this.

My daughter complained that her bottom hurt. So she took her to the doctor sort of hoping that is what it might be. She had written in her diary (which was revealed in court), before this, about this possibility.

I know it does happen a lot. My girlfriend comes home completely strung out from reports of kids who are being molested. But when people in the shelter jump in hook, line, and sinker on the unsubstantiated allegations of people like my ex, and support this kind of fantasy, they are not only doing damage to fathers, they are doing a terrible disservice to the women and children who are being molested, because they're crying wolf and coaching them on how to do it. I hope people will begin to see how it is hurting innocent people's lives.

I have often wondered how many of the homeless men on the streets went through something like I did and didn't have the resources like I had to be able to defend themselves. What if somebody is excited by the plethysmograph pictures but has not, and would not, molest a child? All of this stuff is so unbelievable. Obviously, I'm still having trouble believing it myself.

So you still feel like, in a sense, that you are still being abused and controlled?

Yes, absolutely.

Patricia Overberg of the Valley Oasis Shelter, in an interview with the author, cites the experiences of men like these as a salient factor in making it difficult for a man to leave an abusive relationship:

They have very deep feelings, especially very deep feelings for their children. Because, most of the time, when they do leave, they lose their kids. Fear of ridicule, the macho acceptance of the role of protector and provider come what may, and the fear of losing their children; these are the three things that do make it more difficult, not less difficult, for a man to leave an abusive relationship compared to a woman in the same situation.

The experiences of these men in the judicial and social service systems regarding their children may or may not be typical; however, it is true that many men have heard of these types of incidents. The idea that a man will not be given a fair and equal opportunity in the field of domestic relations law is a pervasive belief. This belief directly affects the ability of the abused man to seek relief under the law.

CALLING THE POLICE

As previously shown, men are less likely than women to report their abuse to authorities. In the British survey by Malcolm George, only 40 percent informed police.

The National Violence Against Women Survey found that men call police only half as often as women, and arrests occur one-third as often.

For those who do summon the courage to call the police, anecdotal evidence suggests that the suppositions of many men about not being treated fairly due to gender may be correct. The complaint of the male victim is often ignored—all over the world. Beryl C. Thurston of Salisbury East, South Australia, has been interviewing a number of Australian male spouse abuse victims. She told of one case in which a man, aged 55, was married for 22 years to an abusive spouse. The violence against him consisted of kicking, punching, and hitting. Thurston contends that there was no evidence that he had ever been violent. During one incident, he did call the police after leaving the house. His wife was not arrested; *he* was.[7]

College student Tim S. told me what happened to him when he called the police after he experienced the most violent incident in his relationship with his live-in girlfriend:

About two months before I moved out, I had gotten home very late, about two in the morning. I was over at a friend's house, who didn't have a phone. There was a pretty heavy snowstorm that day, my car wasn't going anyplace, and the buses were hardly running that night. I tried to get my car going, but I could see that it was a pretty bad idea after slipping and sliding around. Still, that took some time. So I decided to hoof it. I guess his house was two miles from our apartment. I mean, it took awhile and was no fun either.

Anyway, I no sooner put the key in, and opened the door, and she hit me in the head with a frying pan! No warning, no nothin', just bang, right in the head. I got a pretty big gash. I said, "What was that for?" She said it was because she was worried about me! Great, this is the way she shows she's worried about me? I'm really pissed, and I call the police.

Well, this cop shows up, and you could tell, he thinks it's a big joke, you know, smirking. He says, "Well, what'd you let her do that for?" I said, "It's not up to me to stop her." He says something like, "It should have never happened." I told him I wanted to press charges. He said, "There's nothing to press charges on. She's half your size. The judge won't even look at it." He told me I should leave the house for the night. I was upset that it should have to be me that has to leave, but I did. Later, I found out that she had been telling mutual friends that I was very abusive and beat her up all the time. This was really infuriating. But, I figured that the truth would come out eventually, probably with the next boyfriend she has.

Schoolteacher Tom W. called the state police after his wife threw a knife at him and hit him across the shoulder, cutting him. He did request that the police get involved in some way when they showed up:

I asked them to pursue this from a legal standpoint, because I wanted to basically get it resolved and find out what the frustration was. But they said it was too minor, that they really would not pursue it unless the incident would happen again. They did fill out paperwork, because I had called to file a complaint. We were interviewed, together and separately. But, it was dropped right there.

Mark K. says that the police came "at least a dozen times" to his home as the neighbors called them because they heard the yelling and screaming. I asked him what the police did.

Oh, they'd just calm her down, then leave. Usually, they wouldn't do any-thing. The first thing they always wanted to do was go talk to her and find out if she was hurt. They don't care who started it. If she would have said she was hurt, they probably would have hauled me off.

One time we were at her mother's house. We'd been out to dinner and she had a few drinks. Her mom was baby-sitting. So, we went there to pick up the baby. She was getting into one of her freaking-out things, and I told her that we would leave the baby there, and her mom said the same thing. She just got worse, and the cops came and arrested her that time.

How did she attack you that time?

Scratching me on the face, yelling, kicking, hitting. She was screaming so loud that the neighbors, 300 yards down the road, could hear her. That's who called the cops.

What happened when the police came? How did they react?

The first thing the lady cop did when they came is say, "I want to talk to your wife." You could tell, from the tone in her voice, that they first wanted to check to see if she was hurt, a battered wife. Even though I was standing there with blood on my face, and she was not showing any signs of being hurt. As soon as she said that, I just turned and walked away into the house. You could tell she was giving me an attitude. When I walked back out, the lady officer apologized to me. She said, "I'm really sorry. I see your wife is smashed, and I see you have scratches on your face, and I want to take her in."

What did you say?

I said, "No, don't take her in," because she had started calming down by that time; but the police said that under the abuse prevention law they had to arrest her.

What happened next? Was she prosecuted, made to go to classes, or anything like that?

No, nothing like that. I didn't press charges, and no one else did either. The next morning, I went and bailed her out. I did get a letter from the DA [district attorney], a month later, asking me if I wanted to come down and press charges, but I just threw it away.

The experiences of these four men, together with James J.'s experience with the police described earlier in this chapter, anecdotally demonstrate that the police do not react the same way when a man is abused as compared to their reaction when a woman is abused. James J. and Mark K. also mentioned the frustration and difficulty in obtaining a restraining order and having it enforced. The particulars of Mark K.'s case are unique, but his experience in trying to overcome a judge's prejudice is one shared by a number of abused men.

RESTRAINING ORDERS

Mark K. sought such an order after he was severely bitten on the shoulder and chest. He went to his lawyer, who took pictures of his wounds:

> I then went down to file a restraining order, like my lawyer told me to. The lady judge didn't want to see the bites or anything, but she did give me the restraining order.
>
> The next day, Joan [his wife] finds out about it, and she goes to see this same judge. Now get this, she has no marks on her; I never did a damn thing to her. She goes in there, tells the judge that she's in fear for her and the baby's life, that I'm an abusive alcoholic, and so on. The judge vacates my order, gives her full temporary custody of the child, and grants her a restraining order, and the next thing I know, the cops are looking for me to kick me out of the house. My lawyer was furious. [Note: I talked to his lawyer to confirm this story, and *furious* was the word the attorney used to describe his reaction to the judge vacating the prior order without any notification to his client's attorney of record. The attorney got a new hearing for the next day.][8]
>
> I was there at that hearing, with my lawyer. I mean, you could tell, the judge was leading her on. She'd ask, "Well, did he do anything to you in the last 180 days?" I mean, people in the courtroom were shaking their heads. My wife looked down at the ground when she talked; she was just totally unbelievable. It was a real kangaroo court.
>
> The judge kept the restraining order against me in place even though my lawyer brought in police reports and everything about what she had been doing to me. The judge also had the police report she had filed for criminal assault charges, which she told the detectives were false, and that she made it up.

You mean she got the restraining order and requested that criminal charges be brought against you in the same day?

> Right. The police reports were brought in by my lawyer to the next day's hearing, before this judge. After the detectives finished questioning my wife, she admitted that the whole thing was made up, but the judge didn't care. The only thing that got changed was that instead of her getting sole physical child custody, the judge ordered temporary joint physical custody; but I'm kicked out of the house and on notice that if I come around, I'd get arrested.

Okay, then what happened?

> Well, she filed two more false charges. One time, because she didn't have a car [my attorney] didn't want me to do this. I went to the store where we are supposed to make the exchanges in the parking lot, which was O.K. because we could meet to do that, while we both had one week each with the baby. Anyway, I go up there to do the exchange. She started flipping out on me.

I think because I knew that her lawyer had told her that she was going to lose custody, and this was just two days before we were to go to court. The only thing I said to her was, "O.K., I'll see you in court on Friday." Well, this really made her mad, and she says, "I'll fix you."

She calls 911, and the next thing I know, I got three cop cars following me. They arrest me. I asked, "Did she say I hit her?" They said, "No, she said you pointed your finger at her and yelled at her." I was in jail overnight, but she never followed up on the charge of violating the restraining order, and the DA didn't do anything, so it was dropped.

Then, she did it again. This was just recently. She had been calling me all the time, in the middle of the night, while I was at work. One morning, at work, at about four in the morning, she called me up, and I could hear the baby. I said, "What's the baby doing up?" She just says something like that she was just up and didn't say anything about the baby being sick or nothing. I get to the store, at about seven that morning, and this lady comes up and tells me that Joan had taken the baby to the hospital in a rescue unit. I find out at the hospital that the baby has bronchitis. Joan is sitting there with the baby with no clothes on her, just her pants and socks. Joan says, "Well, I don't know how I'm going to get home; I guess I'll just have to hitch-hike." She was trying to make me feel bad and give her a ride. I said, "Well, I need baby stuff from the house, so get in the truck and don't cause any trouble."

I drop her off, get the baby stuff, spend some time with [the baby], and go to work again that night. Now, she had also been calling my baby-sitter, drunk and being abusive and making accusations. I called her and left a message on her machine to stop harassing the baby-sitter, or harassment charges may be filed. That's exactly the way I put it.

The next day she filed another restraining order violation charge against me, saying that I took sex from her the night I dropped her off.

Did she say that you had raped her?

No, she said that I had "practically raped her."

What happened to that criminal charge?

Well, my attorney, on this criminal stuff, says it's about as dead as it can get. I mean, the DA is not going to press charges because her story doesn't match up. She said I was at the house for several hours, but I was at work that night. There's no way I could have been there when she said I was. They really make it hell on a guy trying to fight this stuff.

I have asked a number of prominent domestic relations attorneys from around the United States whether it is more difficult for a man to get a restraining order (as they are called in some jurisdictions) or protective order than it is for a woman in similar circumstances. The replies were quite similar. Portland, Oregon, attorney Ron Johnston, who has been practicing domestic relations law for 15 years, summed it up best:

> It is not as impossible as most men believe. There has been a change in recent years, and more judges are willing to believe that men, too, can be victims of domestic violence and in real danger. However, generally speaking, it is more difficult for a man, and the burden of proof seems to be at a higher standard than for women in the same set of circumstances. Also, generally speaking, in smaller communities and more rural areas, getting a restraining order for a man is more difficult still. I believe many general practice attorneys who don't specialize in domestic relations would hesitate before trying to get a restraining order for a man, whereas there would be no hesitation at all for a woman under the same set of circumstances.

Attorney Johnston mentions the key component for abused men in dealing with the legal system: that most abused men believe the law is not on their side and that getting help via a restraining order is not an option that many consider a possibility. It is, therefore, crucial for abused men to have a place to call to get information for their particular situations. Attorney referrals, dealing with the police, restraining order information, and victim advocacy are all areas in which abused men need help in a timely fashion.

CRISIS LINES

If a crisis line existed for abused men, given their belief system, would they call it? In recounting his story, which focused mainly on child-related issues, James J. has said that he would have called such a line had one existed, and he told of his difficulties in getting help from existing women-only lines. Other men that I interviewed made no effort at all to call existing domestic abuse crises lines because of the assumption that they existed only for women. A significant number of the men I talked to would not have called a crisis line had there been one available. Most cited being too embarrassed to call, or the belief that such situations should always be kept as private as possible. The majority of the men, though, said they would have called such a line had one been available. Steve J. would have called, hoping to get information and help:

> Information on ways to deal with it. Maybe get some help, some ways to deal with it, maybe get her some help…, something. I think it would have been a valuable resource, even if it was just to have somebody neutral to talk to about it.

Tim S., while saying that he never told anyone about the abuse while it was going on, said he would have called an abused men's crisis line:

> To find out what to do, what the options were, how to stop it. I would like to talk to other guys who had the same problem, just to find out that other guys aren't the big pricks that feminists make them out to be. I mean, women want control from men, but they don't have that much control themselves. This thing has made me more suspicious. I don't trust women anymore. I'm afraid of being manipulated....I wasn't that way before.

Tom W. also would have called an abused male crisis line:

> Very definitely. I became very frustrated for many reasons. I lost my vocation. I lost my money. To this day, I'm working three jobs, and I still can't make it financially, what with child support and losing the home. I had no way to pursue it legally. It seems as though I had no one to really turn to. To say, you know, "How can I cope with this?" I felt as though I was out in a boat in the ocean all by myself. I saw so many opportunities for help for women in my situation. I don't deny them that opportunity, because I think there have been quite a few situations, but the other side is, I felt I had been an abused husband, and an abused parent, with really nowhere to turn.

Whether or not the abused male would utilize such a crisis line, the responses of some of the men I talked to indicated that they would have received some comfort just knowing that their problem was not unique. The very existence of a crisis line would help to indicate to these men that they are not alone. For example, at the end of my interview with Mark K., I thanked him for sharing his story and told him that there were millions of men out there who had been attacked by their mates. When I asked him if it helped to know that, he replied: "Really? There are? Yeah, it does help to know that, a lot."

A CHANGING SOCIETY

The exceptional isolation of the abused male may be the characteristic that distinguishes him most from his abused female counterpart. If it is true that men are less likely to seek help with personal problems than women are, it may also be true that many of these abused men (and men in general) have failed to examine their changed role in general societal structures.

The isolation that the abused male experiences is heightened by the increased uncertainty of modem times. Gone are the days when a man could count on his job being there until retirement. The days are also gone, for many people, when only one paycheck is enough. This economic pressure, coupled with the relaxation in social and legal prohibitions against divorce, was the impetus for a necessary change in the workplace to afford equality for women.

The very nature of the work available has also changed. Today the majority of the jobs are in the service sector, and in such fields as computers and high technology, where it is obvious that physical strength carries no extra benefits. The most dangerous and physically demanding jobs are still overwhelmingly held by men. Women simply do not apply for them in any significant numbers. While societal change has been rapid, individual reactions move more slowly. Both men and women are bewildered by the changes in societal defined roles.

Women have developed options in child rearing: part-time work or full-time work. These options are socially acceptable. Male options are more limited. Society still places the highest value (and if women's polls of the ideal husband are any guide, the highest mating value) on a man who is successful financially—the man who can be a good provider. Women have yet to send a message to men that a mate who would make a good homemaker or a good father is as desirable as a mate who is a lawyer or a doctor. Today, of course, there are an increasing number of women who are doctors and lawyers. For the vast majority of males attacked by their mates, societal changes have affected how their mates view them and how they view themselves.

In the next chapter, we will identify the major warning stress points that increase the chances for domestic violence occurring or indicate it already exists. Some people do not know they are in an abusive relationship, or they may suspect they are but need objective confirmation and additional information. Unemployment is one key factor. Men are faced with a new kind of unemployment uncertainty in a society that still values them most for their employment; this prime valuation is shattered in a profound way when they lose their jobs or do not meet their own (or their spouses') expectations for financial success.

The economic pressures that have resulted in a two-income family have profoundly affected men's and women's view of what it means to be a man. If marriage is a partnership and one party is seen, by one or both, as not bringing as much to the partnership, tension is likely to develop. When society does not value males in the family for more than a paycheck, the institution of marriage itself is in danger. The increased divorce rate since the mid-1960s has many causes, but surely part of the cause is this lack of acknowledgment (not to mention appreciation) for the other things that men bring to the family unit.

Is it any wonder that the first question male victims of domestic violence ask is, "What was I supposed to do?" This bewilderment is related to the incidents themselves, but underlying this question is another, even more profound, one: "What am I supposed to be?"

This question may not be limited to only male domestic violence victims, but it does have particular meaning for them. These men are assaulted by their spouses, assaulted by uncertainty in the workplace, and assaulted by the misandry of some feminists—with support in the media. Coupled with the fact that many abused men lose their homes, their possessions, and a continued relationship with their children, it is little wonder that many express a bitterness that may become lifelong.

The cost for these men is obvious. The cost to all of us for failing to recognize their pain, or even laughing at it, is less obvious. It is clear that each time we lose such a man to suicide, alcoholism, unemployment, or depression, we all lose. If society fails to take a stand against all violence and does not recognize the dangerous message such failure transmits to children, efforts against other forms of violence are devalued. Society itself becomes confused and bewildered.

Chapter 3

The Domestic Violence Trap: How to Get Help and Find Freedom from Abuse

There are certain phrases that workers in the domestic violence field hear all too often. From the perpetrator: "I couldn't stop myself." From the victim: "I shouldn't have…, then he/she wouldn't have…" The best answer for the abuser's claim that they had no control—-over their drinking or anger or whatever the reason was for losing control—is this response: "Oh, really? If *60 Minutes* had been filming in your home at that moment, do you think you would have been able to maintain control?" The abuser's response is usually quite different.

I am indebted to Gary Hankins for this clever response to the abuser's usual claim of not being able to prevent the assault. Of particular importance, however, is what Hankins says about victims in his book *Prescription for Anger: Coping with Angry Feelings and Angry People.* This sensitive area is not often discussed. The thing that shelter workers, therapists, social workers, and others must try to help overcome is the feeling of self-blame that many victims have. No one, man or woman, "deserves" to be hit or assaulted by a mate. There is no excuse for violence. This can never be said enough, but the victim may fall into the domestic violence trap by the role they have learned to play. Hankins has concisely defined the victim's role in abusive relationships in his book. He speaks of women as the victims, but there is little difference in the role when it comes to male victims:

> In most battering situations, the woman needs to assume at least partial responsibility for the abuse they receive. Without self-awareness of their own hurtful expressions of anger, these women may be increasing the abuse they

receive....Failure to accept some responsibility for the abusive relationship may lead battered women to become blind to some of the rational options that could help them break out of the abusive cycle. When they deny their anger and turn it inward, irrational options such as suicide or homicide begin to emerge. When battered women try to suppress their anger and rage, it often erupts anyway, despite their best efforts to hide it. Battered women often perpetuate the battering cycle by letting their hurt and anger "leak out" in subtle ways.

Their need to "get even" may be manifested by pouting, giving their mate angry looks, rolling their eyes, contradicting or arguing with their mates, feigning illness to avoid having to interact with them, or "forgetting" to do something they've promised to do (in a passive-aggressive behavior mode).

When a battered woman refuses to accept responsibility for her own behavior she often uses a double standard, claiming that her hurtful retaliations are justified even though her mate's are not....The more frequently couples are abusive with each other, the more habituated they become to the abuse and the more intense it gets. By expressing anger in demoralizing ways, and not moderating the intensity or the duration of it, both the batterer and the battered person perpetuate the destructive cycle of abuse.[1]

Hankins cautions that in cases where the batterer has a severe personality disorder, the abuser considers a mate their "property," and there is little the victim can do to constructively manage their own response or anger.

McNeely and Robinson-Simpson comment in *Social Work* that despite the popular myth that whoever commits these violent acts in the home "must be crazy," the reality is that the overwhelming majority of domestic violence perpetrators are not mentally deranged. This has important implications not only for an understanding by victims and perpetrators but also for law enforcement, social workers, therapists, and others: "Given the magnitude of the problem, it is unlikely that...psychological disturbance is the root of family violence in most instances."[2]

The debate continues among scientists as to what is the proportion of domestic violence perpetrators who suffer from borderline personality disorder and other ills. The total evidence so far, however, suggests that it is not nearly the majority.

The first barrier for victims and perpetrators to overcome, then, is the conviction that anyone who does this type of thing has to be completely out of their mind. This is simply not true for most family violence, so there is the opportunity for people to make an effective change by educating themselves.

RECOGNITION

A typical problem that faces the male victim in particular is denial. A man may feel that he is supposed to be able to take it, that it is "no big deal," or as some victims say, "I can handle it." No one has to take it, and no one should. Abuse *is* a "big deal." It is destructive to every aspect of a person's life. The individual cannot handle it—without some help. Recognition involves identifying what abuse is, and it involves finding out how one responds. See if the types of behavior or reactions listed below are familiar.

- Accepting or giving out rewards after a violent incident. The acceptance rewards may be sexual relations; letting one make a decision; soliciting an opinion on something when opinions are not usually sought; acting in a subservient manner in public or at home; or something else that a partner knows will please, such as an apology, until next time. The rewards the victim gives back usually involve a change, in behavior or doing something else that will please and, it is hoped, pacify the partner.
- Responding to a violent incident by hitting back or acting in some of the passive-aggressive ways that Hankins listed (feigning illness, "forgetting" things).
- If there are children, taking out anger toward the partner on the children.
- Not seeing friends and/or family that the partner does not like or approve of, because to do so might cause a violent episode.
- Having a constant feeling of "walking on eggshells" when at home. Being extremely careful about what one does or says to prevent upsetting the partner.
- Shutting down, by being afraid to give an opinion, avoiding eye contact, finding excuses to go to "private space" (garage, study, yard), finding excuses not to come home. Avoiding the stating of true feelings. Ceasing to participate in family decisions.
- Giving up any voice in how money is spent.
- Drinking or smoking too much or using drugs.
- Having symptoms of depression: losing interest in activities once enjoyed, often feeling sad, feeling worthless or guilty, changes in appetite or weight gain/loss, thoughts of suicide, trouble concentrating, feeling hopeless, being more anxious than usual, digestive problems.

If a person finds many of these reactions to be characteristic of a relationship, there is a problem. Notice that violent acts by a partner were not listed; they will be addressed later. The first step in recognition is finding out how one responds to the threat of violence, or violent acts, from the occasional slap to a severe attack. Next, examine the partner's actions.

- Does the partner block an exit from a room or the house?
- Open personal mail?
- Keep one from seeing friends/family?
- Harshly discipline children when really angry?
- Use name calling?
- Denigrate the other partner in the presence of others?

- Say no one else would want the other?
- Threaten suicide if one were to leave?
- Keep the other partner up late, or wake one up often, even when there is required work or other obligations the next day?
- Often contend the other cannot do anything right?
- Often interrogate about past relationships?
- Have a subservient "mask" in public but act in a very domineering manner at home?
- Get angry at the partner not being sufficiently masculine or demanding enough in dealing with others?

If a number of these factors are true in a relationship, there is a problem. They are characteristics of controlling behavior. Even if just one or two apply, such behavior may extend to other controlling actions in the future. One may have trouble, after looking at these characteristics, deciding what is meant by *often*. The important definition is what the concerned person thinks: If the actions occur often enough to bother, it is too often.

Stress Points

Age. The younger one is, the greater the chances of experiencing domestic violence. Those younger than 30 have a considerably greater probability of occurrence than those 31 to 50 years old and an even greater likelihood of it happening than those older than 50.[3] It is important to remember, however, that these are just probabilities; domestic violence happens to people of all ages.

Religion. If the partners have different religions, the chances of domestic violence are greater.[4]

Employment. If a partner is unemployed, or employed part-time, that person is three times more likely to experience family violence than a person who is employed full-time.[5]

Income. If the family income is below the poverty line, the chance of family violence occurring is 500 percent greater than in an upper-income household.[6] Domestic violence occurs in all kinds of households, however, even among the very wealthy.

Recognizing Physical Violence

Violent acts that are considered domestic violence if they occur include slapping, hitting, kicking, biting, scratching, choking, attempting to burn (cigarette, boiling water), throwing things, and using or attempting to use a weapon of any kind.

The victim should also consider whether they have ever seen a doctor because of injuries sustained, and if the partner tried to discourage or prevent medical attention. Although the surveys of abused men examined in this book are limited in their scope, attacks when asleep seem to be a common factor, as are attempts to kick in the groin. The victim should also consider whether there have been threats of violence. In particular, consider whether there have been death threats, including those that involve getting someone else to carry out an attack.

Personal History

Recognition also means gathering a history for both partners. A family life of a partner that included the parents being physically or emotionally abusive to each other, or to the children, may mean that the partner is more accepting of this behavior in the partner's own relationship. Counseling can be of tremendous value in exploring the family history of both partners. Knowledge in this area helps the partners to understand the background context of the behavior and to find ways to ameliorate the behavior. This does not mean that one should excuse or be accepting of abusive behavior. Those who come from an abusive family background should definitely seek counseling before embarking on a live-in relationship.

Macho Man

Recognition for males includes steps that are somewhat different from those commonly prescribed for female domestic violence victims. The counselors and interviewers presented in this book report some themes for these men that might be called "internal excuses." Some of the most common: "I can fix it and make it better." "I don't want to be weak and admit I can't handle her." "People will think I'm not much of a man if I tell them the real reason we're having problems." "I don't want to be laughed at; no one would believe me."

These internal excuses are understandable, but people do have a right to a home life free from abuse. Being a man does mean being responsible to oneself as well as to others. Putting it all on oneself to handle any crisis will only help set up the time when there is a breakdown. Health, job, and friendships could all suffer. The price to be paid for being a macho "I can handle it" man can be a very high price indeed.

For a man, being afraid to tell others for fear of being laughed at or not being believed are very real issues. These things do happen all too often. There is a risk of unfair treatment. It is important to select carefully whom one decides to confide in.

First Steps

We can only change ourselves; we cannot change others unless they want to change. Perhaps there has been a mutually combative relationship. Both partners have hit each other. Perhaps both come from a family where this is the norm. Now both need to change, but one partner cannot force the other to change. Each must choose to make a commitment toward seeking a new kind of relationship. As odd as it may sound, abusive behavior is often "comfortable" behavior for many. Patterns and habits develop over time in which there is the "high" of an angry scene, the makeup contrite period, and then usually a reward. In other words, the results are known in advance. Breaking out of these long-standing patterns of behavior is not an easy task.

There is a way the stage can be set so real change is more probable. Counseling can help. Men, perhaps more than women, may resist counseling. For some men, there is a feeling that to seek counseling means an admission of weakness, which feeds into the macho and potentially self-destructive "I can handle it" attitude. This also is not an exclusively male reaction; some women express much the same attitude in similar situations.

A technique for overcoming this resistance is to make an analogy with the work environment. At work, when one employee has a disagreement with another employee, the problem is often taken to a third party—another coworker or the supervisor to get another opinion. There is nothing wrong with that. A good work environment encourages a team approach. Certainly, this is better than allowing the disagreement to continue and to get in the way of the job. We all have to work at our personal relationships, too. A counselor will not give an opinion on exactly what should be done; in that sense, it may be different from the job experience. However, good supervisors act in the same way. They will try to get the different viewpoints, ask questions of both parties, try to find some common ground, and help to get both sides to reach an agreement mutually decided upon, not one imposed by authority. A couple's counselor works in much the same way.

Choosing, Obtaining, and Encouraging Counseling

If there is an employee assistance program (EAP) at work, this can be a first stop. Usually, such programs are available only in reasonably large companies. The EAP will help choose an appropriate counselor. Information on why a counselor is being sought is needed so the EAP personnel can make an appropriate referral. If there is no such program available, some creativity is called for, and there may be some difficulty in finding a counselor who understands that men can also be physically abused.

Psychologist Judith Sherven and human behavior expert James Sniechowski are internationally recognized experts in gender reconciliation and relationships. They state that "many, many therapists" show an anti-male bias when it comes to domestic violence. Sherven says it is critical that men get a referral from friends, clergy, or others whom they respect and trust. If such a referral cannot be found, the telephone book can be a start. The abused person should ask pointed questions. The therapist's perspective should be sought, starting with general questions before getting to the particulars of the case. Therapists might be asked questions such as these: "Do you believe men can be battered by their spouses?" "If you do believe that, do you think that men can be victims of the same type of control games that battered women experience?" "Do you think men can be inhibited from leaving a situation that is abusive for many of the same reasons that women might be inhibited?"

Sherven suggests asking about how the therapists pursue the problem and how they go about offering help. The caller should be able to get answers to his questions free of charge on the phone. Sherven says one should try to get a feel for the therapist's personal warmth, care, and compassion. Next, Sherven suggests checking out at least three of the best candidates in one-hour sessions (which are typically not free) to further decide on a final choice. Relevant additional individual questions should be asked that help develop a feel for the therapist's views. If the counselor seems to be leaning toward the viewpoint that when it is the male who is physically abused, the man must have acted in some way that caused the violence, then, obviously, keep looking. The therapy should focus on how to avoid similar situations in the future. It does not matter whether the counselor is male or female. What is important is the counselor's attitude and how comfortable the person seeking help is with the counselor's approach.

Sniechowski says it is also important to be aware of the counselor's general approach to domestic violence:

> First of all, the violence must be stopped. However, under the current orientation toward domestic violence, trying to look at the subtleties of the relationship or assigning responsibilities to both parties is generally called "blaming the victim." In order to protect the person called "the victim" the focus stays fixed, not on the dynamics of both parties that caused the violence but only on the violence itself. Consequently, a state of urgency is inbuilt into the "protect the victim" perspective. Then, when it comes to who's responsible for what, so that both people can learn what they are doing and how they came to be involved, looking at the subtleties, the dynamics, is forbidden. That perpetuates the state of urgency. The violence is the only point. Forceful intervention can be the only method from this perspective, so that personality or character change becomes minimal if possible at all.

> An analogy is that, in war, once the fighting has ceased, it's essential to explore and figure out why both parties were involved. If not, there will

surely be another war—either hot or cold. The cold war is a chronic state of defensive suspicion and paranoia and a chronic state of arms buildup, stored until the next hot war.[7]

If there is a problem in securing private counseling due to low income or lack of insurance coverage, some areas that can be investigated include city/county/state mental health agencies, the United Way Information and Referral service, the Yellow Pages community resources sections for family counseling, and other services that appear to offer family counseling. Community-sourced counseling may not be entirely free, and waiting lists may be long, but most public or nonprofit services offer sliding-scale charges based on income. Some private counselors also offer sliding-scale fee structures. If couple or individual counseling cannot be obtained, there should at least be an attempt to attend an anger management class that may be offered in the area. Individual resistance to considering counseling may be overcome by hearing about others who are dealing with similar experiences and issues. Such a class might be a good first step for many couples to "break the ice" toward discussing areas of concern and seeking additional help.

Primary victims of abuse should probably see the counselor by themselves first. The counselor needs to understand the particular concerns. The spouse can be invited to attend at another time. The counselor's ideas should be sought on nonthreatening ways to encourage this. If the spouse refuses to go, they cannot, of course, be compelled, but there is comfort in knowing that the attempt was made in the best way possible. The abused person should begin the process of locating appropriate counseling and other resources as a first step. There is, however, much that can be done on one's own.

SETTING THE STAGE FOR COUNSELING

What do couples argue about most? Recognizing which areas cause conflict for many people will help increase awareness of potential problem areas in a specific relationship. The top four high-conflict areas for couples who have experienced violence are children, money, sex, and housekeeping. Interestingly, for couples who do not have a violent relationship, polls show that the ranking of these areas would be reversed.[8]

Recognizing that all couples have conflict areas is a healthy way to begin. Whereas it is still very important to seek professional counseling services, there is no reason one partner cannot go ahead and raise concerns in a nonjudgmental way with the other mate.

First, a meeting should be planned with the partner by asking in advance for a convenient time to sit down and discuss something important. It should be a time in which there will be no interruptions and when neither is likely to be tired or stressed. During this meeting, the script might go something like this: "I wanted to talk to you about something that is serious. When you've been upset with me, sometimes you [hit, throw things, etc.]. This really has bothered me. It makes me feel bad. I don't like feeling this way. I'm afraid if you continue to react this way, our relationship will continue to deteriorate. It's really a problem. I'd like to see that it won't happen again. I know we have our disagreements, but that doesn't mean we have to hurt each other. How do you feel when you do this? Does it bother you?"

At this point, the person is mainly looking for recognition that there is a problem with this behavior. Notice there is no blaming. Reframed in the person's own words, the sample script can be useful in explaining how the abused partner feels and in seeking information on how the other feels. It is hoped that the abused partner has already seen a counselor and received guidance on how to assist the spouse in going to counseling together or, alternatively, seeing the counselor on his own. The point of the meeting is to seek a firm commitment by asking for help in solving a serious problem. The counselor's information, or the anger management class information, should be at hand. If the partner agrees to help work on the situation, a positive close would be: "We're agreed then, the appointment will be made tomorrow?" Reminders of the appointment should be made the week and the day before it is scheduled.

CONFLICT MANAGEMENT

Whereas counseling and anger management classes are the most important steps violent couples should take if there is any chance of a continuing relationship, there are some techniques available to resolve conflicts and reduce the chances of a big blowup. We all have times when we are angry. Getting in touch with our own anger and using it in constructive, helpful, healing ways is the subject of Hankins's book. I highly recommend it. Rob Solomon, the author of *Full Esteem Ahead,* teaches conflict management classes. He suggests these techniques for dealing with conflict in a relationship:

1. Assess the real conflicting needs, without getting caught up on the surface. In other words, people often take positions in disagreements and get stuck in them without really looking at what underlies their positions. Communicate your needs clearly, and listen to the other's needs just as clearly.
2. Determine the relative importance of the issues in conflict versus your relationship. Which is more important? Winning the argument or maintaining the relationship? Balance between the two is ideal.
3. Speak up for what you believe is right. Avoiding conflict means you cannot win, and every time you do not try it hurts your self-esteem. Even if you are pretty sure you cannot win, it is important to try.

4. Do not forget the setting when trying to discuss a disagreement. Make sure it is a neutral place, free from distractions, in a safe location.
5. Describe the issue clearly, state how the issue impacts you, and state your feeling about the issue. Ask specifically for the changes you need.
6. Ensure that the other party understands your true and real position by asking for feedback that demonstrates comprehension. Do they she understand what you are talking about?
7. Be prepared to listen to the other person's point of view and to provide feedback to indicate your understanding. Let them know that you understand what they're talking about.
8. Make a plan. Determine what interests each has that can co-exist and which interests are mutually exclusive. Accept what fits and compromise on issues that do not readily mesh.
9. Arrange a specific time to meet to evaluate the results of your attempt to manage the conflict. Make adjustments as needed.[9]

These conflict management techniques can be extremely useful, especially when used in conjunction with anger management classes and counseling to reduce the chances of continued abusive behavior in a relationship. There comes a time, however, when the primary victim must ask themselves whether these efforts have succeeded or if the relationship must end.

STAYING OR LEAVING: HOW TO DECIDE

Lists can be useful tools in helping to organize even very emotional thoughts and feelings. The victim should list all the good things in the relationship in column A. Column B is a list of all the bad things. The two lists should be compared and thought given to what has been written down, then the list should be set aside for a few days. After a pause for reflection, the good and bad things should be put in a most-important to least-important ranking.

The same technique is then used to make two more lists: one to detail the good things that might happen if one leaves the relationship, with column B containing the negative things that might happen if one leaves the partnership. The third list is the reverse, detailing the good things that might happen if one stays, and column B showing the bad things that would likely happen if one stays. After a few days for reflection, the second and third lists are also ranked into most important to least important. It is helpful if these three lists are not put together in one sitting.

These listing exercises may seem somewhat silly, but they can strengthen resolve and help to result in a decision. An independent decision, after perhaps years of being controlled in a number of ways by the other partner, is one of the most difficult tasks the abused person has to face.

Internal Objections to Leaving

"She'll kill herself if I leave." Important questions to consider are: Has she actually threatened to? If she has, could you be around 24 hours of every day? That is what it would take to be absolutely sure of preventing a suicide, if that is what is truly intended. Has counseling been suggested for depression? Has a medical doctor been consulted? Has a suicide crisis line been called and advice considered? Have mutual friends been consulted as to their opinion of this possibility? If she has seen a counselor, what is the counselor's opinion? These bases need to be covered to help answer this internal objection to leaving. It should be noted that while the threat of suicide must be taken seriously, it is a fairly common technique used by abusive spouses as a means to control their mates and ensure that they will stay.

"I'm the responsible one. She'd end up on the street." If you believe your partner does not have the working skills to find employment, help is available. Training could be paid for. A county or state social service agency may provide a number of avenues for assistance. If the partner has been a full-time homemaker, a displaced homemaker program may be available in the area. Spousal support may be a part of a legal separation or divorce, and an attorney could be consulted as to the details of the likely amount. The bottom line is that help is available.

There are nearly unlimited areas for which the partner who is leaving might feel responsible. As noted before, one partner cannot help the other if they will not accept the help. There are resources. If it is a drinking or drug problem, Alcoholics Anonymous, local treatment centers, and chemical dependency counselors are all areas that could be investigated. The help of family and friends could also be sought.

The chief internal objection to leaving the abusive partner may indeed be guilt over abdicating one's own sense of responsibility and commitment to the partnership and the household. This involves the underlying reason behind the more openly stated one: not leaving because of practical economic matters. The partner who leaves an abusive relationship can find solace in some measure for these understandable feelings of guilt if they have done everything reasonably possible to secure needed help. Comfort may also be found in the possibility that the former partner may be less likely to be involved in another abusive relationship. Self-blame for leaving an abusive situation when all avenues for constructive change have failed cannot be entirely avoided for many people. Time and distance will help. The most important thing is not to lose faith in relationships but to make absolutely certain that there is no involvement in another abusive relationship.

"But I still love her." Yes, this is important, but sometimes the price of love is too high.

Examine the lists again. The question to ask is if the abused partner is willing to pay the necessary price to remain in the relationship. If one is in a controlling and abusive relationship, and all possible avenues for help for both partners have been explored, and the abusive behavior continues, there is only one choice: *Leave!*

External Objections to Leaving

"What about the children?" Although direct help for abused men may be limited (few regular support groups exist), most men's rights groups in the United States do have a long history of dealing with custody and visitation issues. Contacting a local group could prove beneficial insofar as attorney referrals and legal consumer information. Some groups have book lists and information on divorced parenting classes that will help both child and parent through the separation process. In a growing number of counties in the United States, divorced parenting class is now mandatory for both partners after divorce papers are filed. The keys to a less traumatic separation for both child and parent are information, education, and careful planning.

Staying out of the courthouse should be a prime consideration. A legal battle over custody or visitation greatly increases the chance that the children will be harmed in the process and increases the chance for a battle continuing between former spouses that may result in partial or full loss of a relationship between one of the parents and the children.

Mediation

The best alternative to court is mediation. In certain counties in the United States, mediation may be mandated for custody or visitation disputes once divorce papers are filed. One need not wait for a mandatory session, as a private mediator can be hired. Inquire if the mediator is a member of the American Academy of Family Mediators, which will help assure the individual's training. The court system may also offer mediation sessions even when they are not mandatory. A family mediator can help settle all matters relating to custody and visitation outside of court. Once an agreement is reached, it is simply put into legal language and filed. The process is much less expensive than attorney fees and court costs, and it greatly increases the chance of a smoother separation, because the mediator seeks to have both partners be as satisfied as possible with the result. The mediator also helps to ensure a continued relationship with the children for both parents.

Financial Support

Child support is set in the United States by federally mandated state guidelines. Call the office of child support enforcement to obtain a copy of the guidelines, or they are most commonly available through a state Web site. Whether one becomes a custodial parent, a noncustodial parent, or a joint-custody parent, it helps to know in advance how things will look financially.

Visitation

Even when there is joint physical custody, visitation is an important issue. The key to a continued parental relationship and to a separation that is less stressful for the children is advance planning. Emergency restraining or protective orders often deal with visitation in a general way, and what seems temporary often has a way of becoming permanent under law. Judges do not like to force children through too many changes in residence or lifestyle.

Many court jurisdictions specifically define what is meant by "reasonable visitation." It is important to obtain a copy of the court's visitation guidelines before a partner leaves the home. There may be special considerations that need to be addressed in even a first hearing. *Vague and general final visitation orders should especially be avoided by a partner leaving an abusive situation.* Precisely set times for pickup and delivery, prohibitions against verbal abuse of the other parent in the presence of the children, and remedies or consequences for late pickups or nondelivery are some of the issues that should be addressed. Supervised visitation should be considered in cases of child abuse or threat of child abduction. Attention to the long term should be given in the beginning in order to make return trips to court less likely.

Separating parents' classes, books on making separation less traumatic for the child, the advice of an attorney, legal consumer groups, and mediation are all helpful avenues to be used. The information gleaned will help to construct a workable visitation arrangement. Use the time between a temporary order and a final one to constructively gather information and examples that can be applied to an individual situation.

While visitation is not often easy for the custodial or the noncustodial parent, parents who separate due to domestic violence need to be especially careful not to use the child as a weapon against one another. A large body of research suggests that parental separation in itself can be healthy for the child who benefits by the removal from partner acrimony but that the child can be harmed by continued conflict after separation, especially when drawn into the arguments by being asked to take sides and other reprehensible demands. Children can also be damaged by the loss of a continued relationship with one of the parents. Custody is an adult decision; visitation and adequate financial support are a child's rights.

The partner who separates from an abusive relationship may justifiably resent and resist continued contact with the other partner for the purposes of visitation. There are alternatives to face-to-face contact, such as exchanges through a third party. Supervised or monitored exchanges can be made, or they can be conducted in a public place such as a shopping mall or police department parking lot. Given time, adequate structure, and safeguards, visitation can take place without undue stress for parents or children.

Parents who attempt to block or impede visitation may face legal challenges. For partners who have left an abusive situation, it is vitally important that the child not be drawn into old emotional issues or be used as a means to try to control the former partner. For men, who face a statistically greater likelihood of being noncustodial parents, the abusive former partner may continue to try to establish control through visitation blocking, denial, or using the bait of increased visitation in exchange for favors. Anyone who is denied visitation rights needs to discuss the situation with an attorney. The most important item in any such case is proof; a witness to the denial of court-ordered visitation is vital. It is also important for the child that the noncustodial parent take care not to give up on visitation attempts or fall into the trap of denigrating the former partner to the child. A continued demonstration of caring is vital for the child's self-esteem. Denouncing the other parent to the child usually backfires, by forcing the child to defend that parent or take on an unfair adult role as a mediator. Support groups for children of separated parents are available in some school districts and provide an opportunity to share common visitation problems and other issues with peers under a counselor's guidance. Such groups are particularly valuable for a child without siblings.

TAKING THE BIG STEP TO LEAVE

Many of the professionals and volunteers who work with battered spouses report the common phenomenon of remaining past the reasonable expectation of any improvement. The abused spouse may live with the perpetrator for years, until there is the "last straw," which may not be an incident that is particularly more violent than previous ones but seems to be a final, strong internal recognition of the futility of trying to change the other person.

This emotional moment is necessary but has its dangers. Leaving the household in a hurry may have long-term adverse consequences. The phrase "possession is nine-tenths of the law" has particular meaning in domestic relations cases. Leaving valued material possessions in the hands of a vindictive spouse could result in their being damaged, sold, or destroyed. Even if the victim believes the children are not in danger, leaving them with the former mate may greatly limit the chances of legal custody later.

If the victim of abuse is still undecided about leaving or waiting for that last-straw incident, an emergency exit plan should be drawn up. Such a plan is necessary to ensure a safe temporary haven from a real threat of death or abuse. Unfortunately, for the male victim, domestic violence shelters are not an option except in a very few places, so planning is especially necessary to prearrange a place to stay on an immediate basis, probably with a relative or friend who will readily accept both the victim and the children. Money adequate for transportation and at least some nights of commercial lodging should be set aside privately. Supplies and clothing adequate for children and self should be preidentified, and if one needs to return home to gather belongings, the police should be asked to provide protection.

Restraining Orders

The restraining/protective order removes an abusive partner from the home. The victim and any children stay. It will need to be proven in a hearing (usually within two weeks) that both parties attend that there has been domestic violence. A man may face a higher standard of proof that he is the primary victim. It is critical for both men and women victims to prepare for a restraining order before one is actually sought. The first step is to go to the courthouse and obtain information about how the restraining or protective order process works. Emergency restraining order hearings with a judge are usually limited to certain times of the day. These hearings are most often very brief. The victim may get assistance in some localities with a court-appointed advocate. Such an advocate should prove valuable in convincing the judge that the case is serious enough to warrant an emergency temporary order. The victim may need time to schedule an appointment with the advocate in advance of the emergency hearing.

If the police have responded to incidents of domestic violence at the household in the past, copies of those reports need to be obtained and presented at the emergency temporary restraining order hearing and again at the hearing in which the order is extended, changed, or not allowed to continue. The victim needs to be prepared to assist their attorney (or without an attorney, to help inform the judge) with testimony or credible documentation from other household members, relatives, friends, and acquaintances who have witnessed, seen the results of, or can offer corroborating evidence of domestic violence.

Any hospital or physician medical records about injuries should be introduced. If there are observable injuries, photographs of the injuries should be taken and a credible witness or documentation provided as to the circumstances of the pictures.

Thousands of restraining orders are obtained every day in the United States, and the majority are granted without the assistance of an attorney. The male victim, however, faces obstacles unique to his gender. Advice as to which judge and/or advocate may be more understanding of his plight could be crucial. Knowledge of personnel in the district attorney's office if criminal charges are sought may also be vital. The male victim in particular should seek out an attorney in advance of the need. Finding an attorney who has had prior experience successfully representing male abuse victims will likely take some extended effort, and in some localities, an attorney with prior experience in such cases may not exist. It may take some time to locate a person with adequate expertise in domestic relations law who will not hesitate to be a strong advocate and who is aware of any sexism in the system.

GOING BACK

Restraining orders and criminal charges are often dropped or ignored by a domestic violence victim following a reconciliation with the partner. The victim is relying on promises that the abuse won't happen again. The dynamic of domestic violence feeds on the regrets of both victim and perpetrator, and there can be no guarantee that there will not be a repeat of a violent episode. The victim should not rely on promises. They should demand specific steps before considering returning. These steps should at a minimum include anger management classes and counseling. If alcohol or drug abuse is part of the situation, a comprehensive and completed treatment program should be required.

The primary physical abuse victim should not neglect their own specific steps before considering returning. Gathering information through reading and from others about domestic violence should be a priority, including resources directed at abused women, because of the similarities previously discussed. Counseling to better understand the victim's role in an abusive situation is necessary, not only to ensure that one is prepared to break out of roles and patterns of behavior that contribute to a lack of self-esteem typical of abuse victims, but also to help identify factors that may contribute to seeking relationships based on domestic violence in the future.

If the victim does return after specific conditions are met, they should still be prepared to act quickly with the previously described emergency exit plan and other steps in place. There must be no acceptance of being physically or verbally abused again. One more abusive act must be the last, last straw. Male victims tend to be particularly dismissive of so-called minor acts, but it does not matter if he has been "not hardly hurt" or has had much worse happen to him on the athletic playing field. It is abuse when it comes from one's mate. The victim must wrest control from his mate and give it to himself. He must not return to or accept old dysfunctional patterns of behavior in the relationship. Support in leaving does exist. The victim must accept the responsibility and task of finding that support and taking the necessary step of never returning to this or any other abusive relationship again.

FINDING SUPPORT

The best support starts with self-help. While this does not mean that one should not seek out counselors or others, it does mean that control can be regained. Getting back in control means not accepting or reinforcing all the bad things the mate has said about the victim's character, habits, abilities, and interests.

This can start with an examination of feelings about self-worth by listing the attributes, qualities, and good deeds that make one a worthwhile person. If the abuse has been long-standing, there may be some difficulty in coming up with much; this is all right, and the list can start with just a few basic things. Examples could include: (1) I'm on time for appointments; (2) I'm kind to children and animals; (3) I don't drink too much; (4) I helped another person today by—.

No attempt should be made to complete the list in one day, or in any specified time period. The idea is to write something down every day. When something is added, the entire list can be read again. There is no "finish" to this exercise. It can be a lifelong process to discover new good qualities about oneself. This simple but powerful exercise can begin the process of strengthening damaged self-esteem.

Restoration of the personal image is going to take some time and work. This cannot be accomplished unless the abused person takes stock of the opportunities available and personally starts the process.

Friends and Family

Victims of domestic violence are generally uncomfortable discussing this aspect of their lives with someone else. It is often the case that friends and family are the last to know. Letting a more casual acquaintance or coworker know is more threatening for some but easier than telling friends and family for others. Some never share this hidden side of their family life with anyone.

The male victim faces particular strictures in revealing to others. The lack of public recognition of the problem for men adds to the feeling of isolation and self-blame for a situation that seems personally unique or at least very rare. The lack of local nonprofit crisis lines to discuss issues with a neutral informed party is particularly cruel. The male victim is left to his own devices.

There is opportunity for the man, by turning to his own essential maleness—putting on a "hero hat"—and accepting a challenge, to battle the fear of rejection. In one sense, sharing his story with another is a heroic act of selflessness; through the sharing of such stories, other abused men can learn they are not alone. The great risk is being laughed at, treated dismissively or derisively, or being told in effect that he is a "wimp" for not using a possibly greater physical strength to strike back.

Deception is generally not a healthy practice, but for men who may have trouble getting started with that one essential first person, it may be necessary. The male victim can tell the story exactly as it occurred, including all the important details, but pretend it happened to a female close acquaintance or friend. He can accept and listen to the other's reaction. Then he can explain that it wasn't a woman experiencing this abuse; it was a man—himself. This trick does indeed set the stage for a real "listening post" not burdened by sexism.

The male victim, just like the female victim, deserves and needs a nonjudgmental person to share his story with. Both genders can experience difficulty obtaining the kind of help they need. They may be blamed for leaving or for staying so long. They may be expected to be completely happy right away, instead of still feeling lonely and depressed. There may be attempts to be overprotected by family. The family needs to understand that any live-in arrangement is temporary and help is needed to regain independence.

Finding and Affirming Support through Regained Control

One reason it is difficult for an abused person to find a friend or family member to confide in is because to do so is an admission of loss of control over one's life. Abused husband Don W. probably said it best: "She had all the power. I had nothing. It was a very bizarre situation. It's not that I let her have it; she just took it. The only thing I could do was battle her physically, and I refused to do it." Part of gaining control and supporting oneself by accepting help means accepting that powerlessness. When counseling, discussion, ignoring the behavior, or even some form of retaliation have all failed to stop the abuse, the feeling of having no personal power is acute.

Personal guilt should not be assigned for being unable to change the other person. Changing the situation is the only thing the abused person can control. Financial obstacles to leaving may be daunting, but they are less likely to be overcome without some assistance from friends, family, or other resources. Not revealing the real reason for leaving or intending to leave is deceptive and does not sufficiently convey the urgency of the need. Such deception may delay proper help and tends to furnish self-destructive ammunition in failing to confront and recognize core relationship issues. Only in accepting a problem as one we live with can we find the means to deal with it constructively. Unless this step is taken, the problem is likely to occur again. Freedom from abuse may be short-lived unless acceptance, control, and outside help are all actively sought.

CELEBRATING AND AFFIRMING FREEDOM
FROM ABUSE

The abused person who has left the relationship is not free from all problems. To give but one example, many experience guilt related to feeling that they gave up on responsibilities and commitments. These are understandable and can be worked through with time and counseling.

It is imperative, however, that the abused person not stand in harsh judgment of himself. A checklist of positive qualities about his character and good actions as well as what has been gained by leaving the abuse is very helpful. Abused men and women often have doubts about themselves sexually. They have often been told repeatedly they are unattractive or would not be appealing to others. These kinds of "knockdowns" and others can now be left behind.

The abused person often feels that they were living with a "crazy person" and suffered many worries about whether the partner would harm themselves or others. Freedom from constant confrontation, "walking on eggshells," hiding at work, and being afraid of embarrassing public scenes are common concerns that can now be left behind. If there are children involved, some of these problems may occur again, but at least they will be less frequent.

Affirmation of the good things that open up for the person now free from abuse is extremely important. Some of the affirmation opportunities the abused person should recognize include the chance to feel affectionate again, to not be depressed, to try new things, to meet new people, to talk honestly with others, and to have one's feelings respected.

Another positive way to celebrate, affirm, and improve self-esteem is to give self-rewards. The most long-lasting rewards are those that focus on self-improvement and helping others. The abused person can start with accomplishing small goals and work toward larger ones. Individual circumstances vary, but perhaps there is a book you have always wanted to read, or you have a goal of exercising more, reviving or starting a hobby, or taking a trip. Whatever your case may be, one small accomplishment can lead to another. For the abused male in particular, contacting other men with similar issues and concerns is "other directed" and in the larger picture would greatly benefit others, both men and women, because support groups and other positive steps might result.

Celebrating and affirming freedom from abuse also means seeking out opportunities for fun. Try something different through confronting and overcoming the fear of being alone. Go to the zoo, a museum, an art gallery (a great way to meet new people), take in a play, give a party, take a hot air balloon ride—anything that is new or something not done in a long time has to be tried in order to help overcome understandable fears that can lead to isolation and potentially further dependence on the same type of relationship just escaped. As American patriot and adventurer Davy Crockett said, "Be sure you're right, then go ahead!"

THE MALE DIFFERENCE

The situation of the abused male in the relationship dynamic, and of the issues that must be confronted, is more similar to his female counterpart than it is different. I have attempted to point out the similarities in this chapter as well as some of the differences. One major difference is an extreme emphasis on the perceptions of others. For this reason, and because it involves a series of incidents not widely known, it is instructive to learn what the public perception has been historically and to learn what resistance or encouragement has occurred in recognizing the issue of the abused male who has been assaulted by his mate as a significant social problem. The next chapter explores the history of debate on the subject, examines media and social service influences, and helps to explain why individual abused men currently face unique obstacles.

For listings of contact groups, see Selected Resources following the Selected Bibliography.

Chapter 4

Resistance and Acceptance: The Challenge to Understanding

In previous chapters, we explored some key obstacles to obtaining assistance for abused men. Disbelief and ridicule are two areas that most often set the male victim apart from his female counterpart. We have seen that the male victim has few resources and finds little support among public agencies or in the media, which in turn increase his isolation. Resistance to the concept of a male victim of domestic violence is high and, in some instances, virulent. To understand the current status of men who find themselves in this situation, it is helpful to examine both negative and positive reactions and the parameters of the debate.

As mentioned in the Introduction, I expected this book to result in controversy. Indeed, it was more a certainty than an expectation, given what has happened to a number of others who have publicly examined this issue. There have been shootings, bomb threats, death threats (even against children), career threats and actions, and attempted character assassinations. The expectation that this book would be controversial has been born out. In the 10 years since it was first published, many attitudes have changed, and in many cases, turned into action, but there is still resistance.

It perhaps confirms Schoepenhauer's dictum: "All truth goes through three stages. First, it's ridiculed; next, it's violently opposed; third, it's generally recognized as being true."

It is helpful, then, to look at what has happened in the past, to recognize the ridicule and the violent opposition, before examining what has changed in the past 10 years.

THE ACADEMIC DEBATE

One example is the case of Suzanne Steinmetz, currently a professor at Indiana University. While at the University of Delaware, she coauthored *Behind Closed Doors: Violence in the American Family*. This book was one of the first to explore the entire range of family violence; it was widely praised, it was used as support for women's groups, and not much controversy came about as a result of it. The work was based on the 1975 National Family Violence Surveys (NFVS) supported in part by funding from the National Institute of Mental Health and led by Murray Straus and Richard Gelles at the University of New Hampshire Family Research Laboratory. This first survey was used extensively to significantly raise official estimates of the degree of domestic violence against women in the United States and served as a basis for projections of its pervasiveness throughout the world. Although information was given on the amount and depth of violence by women against their mates, this aspect of the work was mainly ignored.

In 1977, Steinmetz submitted an article based on the survey to *Victimology* entitled "The Battered Husband Syndrome."[1] The popular press ignored the article at first, but some feminists brought it to their attention by denouncing it. Steinmetz, in an interview with me, said: "If they hadn't attempted to suppress it, it probably wouldn't have gotten any attention."

> I was on the *Donahue* show several times, and we must have gotten 7,000 pieces of mail. It came in bags. The university didn't know what to do with it. I didn't know what to do with it. We answered what we could, usually the very worst cases that seemed to need the most attention, and we gave them what referral help we could. I mean, I'm not an attorney, just a researcher. It was overwhelming. A large proportion of the mail was from women, seeking help for their battering problem against their spouses. They told of being turned away or being offered no help when they called a crisis line or shelter. I also got a lot of letters from second wives telling what had happened to their husbands, and a lot of letters from battered men as well.[2]

While Steinmetz was getting this reaction from the public at large after her *Donahue* appearances, some colleagues in the academic community were hard at work. Three professors at separate universities and a director of an abused women's coalition wrote a scathing rebuttal attack on her article in *Victimology*. Despite Steinmetz's statement in her conclusion, "This paper is not intended to de-emphasize the importance of providing services to beaten wives," the critics feared that this was exactly what she was doing.

> If the misrepresentation of data in this article had been limited to its publication in this journal, its effect would have been serious, but correctable

by debate among scholars. However, the "findings" of Dr. Steinmetz have received wide attention in newspaper reports, in family advice columns, and from congresspersons considering legislation about family violence. It may have led to a reduction in public support for programs to aid battered wives, and in all of these, Steinmetz' NIMH (National Institute of Mental Health) funding is used to lend credibility to her thesis.[3]

Since the letter to *Victimology* is four pages long, it is not practical to reprint it here; however, the writers used language unusual for an academic critique, stating that they were "frankly disturbed by the quality of the scholarship," and they described her paper as "a serious cause for alarm."

Steinmetz pointed out that NIMH did not support the research writing for the article, although it did provide support for the NFVS. She countered by saying the critics were comparing apples to oranges in criticizing the data; that is, while it is true that wives are injured in greater numbers by their husbands, the average violence scores show wives to be slightly more likely to resort to violence than husbands. Her critics also denounced her for using the word *often* in describing the level of physical violence used by wives against husbands. Steinmetz said since one-third of the cases involved wife-initiated violence against husbands "'often' is an appropriate adverb."

More important than issues over data and the choice of words is the tone used by the academic critics. They reprinted a letter from an abused women's coalition: "Your 'even-handed' research gives people the opportunity to quibble over numbers and allows them to ignore the real suffering and lack of alternatives in women's lives." The three professors added, "It is beyond the scope of our critique to consider the responsibility of social scientists to accurately represent data in scholarly articles and to the public....But the combination of the social importance of the topic and the wide dissemination of the 'findings' poses a most serious issue for our profession."

Steinmetz had a one-page reply, the concluding statement of which went beyond the data debate (after she defended the numbers she used) and addressed what was at the heart of her critics' concern that bringing up these numbers might hurt services to battered women:

> My goal...was to assemble as much data as possible on a virtually ignored topic; provide historical examples supporting the long existence of this phenomenon, thus refuting the claim that husband abuse is the result of the women's movement, ERA [Equal Rights Amendment], women's increasing aggressiveness, etc.; and to propose some possible explanations for discrepancies between these findings and earlier studies. Any goals beyond these are fantasies in the minds of my critics. I am disturbed, however, by my critics' convoluted "logic" and by the great extent they have gone to locate "errors"

in an attempt to discredit the findings. Their comments regarding my selec-
tivity in "approving" of certain examples or my failure to note that wives
may have been provoked into abusing their husbands are uncomfortably
similar to the responses which greeted those reporting on wife abuse only a
few years ago.[4]

What happened to Steinmetz later, however, made the academic debate seem
mild. As she explained in an interview with me:

> In an attempt to try to keep me from speaking, I had thinly veiled threats
> put on me. I was speaking at an American Civil Liberties Union conference
> [a champion of free speech concerns], and they received threats. They were
> told if they allowed me to speak, the place would be bombed.
>
> Every female faculty member of the University of Delaware was called and
> told that if they wanted to preserve women's rights, they needed to do every-
> thing possible to keep me from being promoted. The people doing this were
> what I would call radical-feminist groupies. That is, they weren't mainstream
> feminists, or even that directly involved, but took what one feminist group
> spokesperson said, about keeping me from being noticed, to the extreme.
>
> The faculty members ignored this. In fact, I didn't even learn about the
> calls until years later. They knew it wasn't true. They knew of my work in
> helping to set up some of the first abused women's shelters in Delaware.
> They just ignored it.
>
> I also received a couple of phone calls saying it wouldn't be safe for my
> children to go out. At the time, because of stupidity, naïveté or false bravado,
> I'm not sure which, I didn't put much stock in it because I knew these peo-
> ple. People who would make outrageous statements to get press, but who
> I didn't really believe in my heart were violent people. But some of their fol-
> lowers didn't have common sense.
>
> The whole thing was fairly short-lived, about a year. Since then, except for
> snide comments by a few critics in academia, who must have nothing better
> to do, there hasn't been much.
>
> Interestingly enough, much later, about three years ago, there was a very
> positive thing that happened, although it started out like some of the other
> things from years ago. I was told before giving an address at a Canadian uni-
> versity I would have major problems by one group of radical women. They
> wrote to the college president and said I should be stopped from coming to
> speak.
>
> Well, I went to speak anyway, of course. I'm giving my speech; I notice
> this group of women shaking their heads and agreeing with me. Because
> I'm pointing out that the bottom line is that women get the short end of
> the stick anyway. When we say women can't possibly be violent, she must
> have done it for some reason, it's nothing, it's no big deal, let's ignore it, and
> so on, we are in essence denying women services. When a man beats up a

woman, right away he's put in a program for batterers. He's given support. He's helped to deal with his problems. He's also sometimes sent to jail. But when a woman does it, it's passed off as, "No big deal, honey. He probably deserved it. Now go home." No one gives her support. No one says, "Gosh, if you're acting in this way, you might be troubled." Even to the point where women come in and ask for help, they're told, "Oh it's not a problem; it's his problem. Don't worry about it."

I was making the point in this speech that no matter how you cut it, even in a case where the man is the victim of the abuse, the system has denied women any services so that they wouldn't do this again or so that they might feel in control. I don't know how many service providers have called me up and told me how they had to turn these women away because they don't know what to do—they don't have any services for them.

In many cases, the radical feminists running the shelter would put a political twist on things. They would tell these women, "He must have done something." When a woman asks for help, and is told that she doesn't have a problem, that it's her mate's fault, it is very similar to what was happening in the 1950s and 1960s to abused women.

That's when women were very depressed, and they had a lot of clinical depression. They couldn't explain why. The doctor would say, "Oh, honey, there's nothing wrong with you. You've got a good husband. It's all in your head." Society was saying, "Your problem isn't real."

After the speech, I asked my academic colleagues over dinner where the radical women's group was that was going to shout me down and prevent me from speaking. They told me it was the group sitting over in one corner that was agreeing with what I was saying, and asking questions, and saying how wonderful it was.

That evening, we had a very unusual (for an academic speech) open-to-the-public forum. It was like what we used to see in the early years when we did battered women's events. Men were running up to the microphone and talking about how they had been abused. Women were jumping up and comforting them. Women were jumping up and talking about how they abused their husband, and they felt so bad, and didn't know where to turn, and another woman would jump up and comfort her. Another man would get up and tell how he had been abused, and a woman or a man would comfort him, like that…, through most of the evening. I felt real awkward. I'm not used to things like that. I felt like I was at a revival or something.

I think that, for whatever reason, I must have hit some sort of chord that made real good sense even to the radical feminists, at least in terms of women being denied services by denying the problem.

I also pointed out that I have testified as an expert for battered women in cases where they have killed or attempted to kill their husbands, that is, women who have been severely battered over a length of time. You do try to emphasize the number of women who have been in this situation. You do try to make the case that this is not unique. You do give evidence to support someone who in desperation, in order to save her life, in a self-defense mode, kills or tries to kill her husband.

That is very different, however, from an academic study in presenting findings. I have real problems with people who say, "Well, if a woman can be violent, then there's no credibility in the battered woman syndrome." Well, that's bull. That's like saying that because some women or men can be violent, then all women or men should be able to protect themselves. We know that's not true; it's not logical.

I think when the radical women's group wrote to keep me from speaking at this university, they viewed me as someone with horns. When people don't know the issue, you get defined as someone with a political agenda. They didn't really know why I should be prevented from talking, and when they actually heard my message, it made sense.

What happened to me [in terms of negative reaction] is nothing, trust me, compared to what Murray Straus has gone through. He always says I had it worse, but I don't think so. I think it's an interesting gender thing probably.

I have been at meetings where he was, and if people had said to me the things that were said to him in a public academic setting...I don't know, I would have been upset.

He always passed it off as no big deal. He's had women academics come up to him and almost physically accost him in the hall because they've been so angry. I guess that's part of this whole thing, that we assume men can take it and women can't. I think he had it much worse than I did.[5]

Murray Straus has been past president of the National Council on Family Relations, past president of the Eastern Sociological Society, a member of the American Association for the Advancement of Science, and president of the Society for the Study of Social Problems. He has won the Ernest W. Burgess Award from the National Council on Family Relations for outstanding research on the family; the National Family Violence Surveys that he and Richard Gelles began have been recognized as the most reliable instrument for measuring domestic violence. This work is supported by the University of New Hampshire and made possible in part by grants from the National Institute of Mental Health.

Straus has been heckled and booed and has been prevented from speaking at several forums on college campuses. He was picketed several times. He was subjected to a planned walkout during his presidential address to the Society for the Study of Social Problems. At his university, there was a telephone campaign accusing him of being a misogynist and of sexually harassing students. Although his name has been put forward several times to be nominated for office in the American Sociological Association, he has never actually been nominated; he suspects this is due to his reports about male victims of domestic violence. The type of attacks he has endured is illustrated in a series of events and press reports involving a Canadian spokesperson for battered women.

Pat Marshall was executive director of the Canadian Panel on Violence against Women and executive director of the Toronto Action Committee on Public Violence against Women and Children. She spoke to a reporter for *Toronto Life* in her capacity as director of the government-funded panel on Violence against Women. When asked about the work of Murray Straus, she stated:

> I know Murray. I was speaking at an international conference a few years ago in Jerusalem....Was introduced to a woman....I have never met a woman who looked so victimized. Never in my whole life. By coincidence it turned out to be Murray Straus's wife. I have never met somebody who was trying so desperately to be invisible in the space that she occupied. I mean, it was just dramatic.[6]

Marshall, according to the reporter, repeated the allegation that Straus had sexually harassed students. She did not respond to any questions about the validity of the work of Straus and other researchers at the Family Research Laboratory in New Hampshire. Marshall, when asked about the work of Straus during her 1991 stint as panel chair, repeated similar negative claims around Canada, according to the *Toronto Life* report.

The reporter called Straus to ask about these claims. Straus denied sexually harassing students, and he noted that while the university had received several complaints from outsiders in the past, it had found no cause for action or even investigation. As to beating his former wife, he suggested the reporter talk to her. The reporter did so, and she confirmed that in 40 years of marriage her husband, from whom she is now divorced, had never struck her. (Though I hesitated to repeat this type of allegation, it is necessary to do so in order to demonstrate the depths of some of the attempts of those with "official" status to discredit Straus.) When Straus complained to Canadian government officials about the Marshall remarks, she wrote a letter of apology; however, in the apology she claimed she never made the remarks attributed to her by the reporter and heard publicly by numerous people. Straus decided to take no legal action.

In Straus's interview with me, I found Steinmetz's characterization of his response to years of attacks to be an accurate one. He passes it off as no big deal and as coming with the territory. I doubt, however, whether many other academics have been subjected to the kind of harassment and blatant attempts at intimidation that he has had to experience.

It is important to remember that the work of Straus and others at the Family Research Laboratory focuses on domestic violence against men in only a minor way. The majority of the work has generated little controversy and is widely accepted and referred to. Indeed, as pointed out earlier, the results developed are the main source cited by advocates for battered women. The work also examines numerous other areas of family violence and discord.

Despite this, Straus has had to write several papers defending his and others' work in this one area. While he is dismissive of the personal attacks, he has not been reluctant to defend the research in academic papers:

> These critics argue that the family violence approach and the feminist approach are irreconcilable. On the contrary, what is irreconcilable are these critics erroneous depiction of family violence research as ignoring gender and power and their narrow and erroneous depiction of feminism....I [include] the possibility that [errors that are repeated often enough] are deliberate distortions intended to discredit the scientific findings by discrediting the researchers whose studies revealed the equal rates of assault. Many of the critics state or imply that family violence researchers ignore the fact that male violence results in more injury than does female violence. This is truly incredible, because that very point has been emphasized in every one of my books and papers on this issue since the 1970s. The implication is that family violence researchers want to give priority to violence by women, whereas my publications over many years have consistently stated the opposite. The claim is that I misrepresent the nature of marriage as a partnership of equals. In fact, a central focus of my research since the early 1970s has been studies showing male dominance and its pernicious effects, including violence against women....Almost every time that critics use the phrase, "feminists argue," it can be replaced by citations to publications in which "Straus argues." These feminist issues include institutionalized male power, cultural norms legitimating male violence against women, and economic inequality between men and women that locks women into violent marriages. These contributions were widely cited until I published "politically incorrect" data on violence by women and was therefore excommunicated from feminist ranks. However, I remain one of the faithful, and have never accepted the excommunication....Perhaps the most important conceptual error is the belief that the Conflict Tactics Scale [CTS] is deficient because it does not measure the consequences of physical assault [such as physical and emotional injury], or the causes [such as a desire to dominate]. This is akin to thinking that a spelling test is inadequate because it does not measure why a child spells badly, or does not measure possible explanations of poor spelling. The concentration of the CTS on [specific kinds and severity of] acts of physical assault is deliberate and one of its strengths.

The attacks on the CTS are examples of blaming the messenger for the bad news. Moreover, no matter what one thinks of the CTS, at least four studies (that number has vastly increased since then) that did not use the

CTS also found roughly equal rates of violence by women. It is almost beyond belief that some critics can ignore or dismiss these studies. Perhaps even more serious is the implied excusing of assaults by women because they result from frustration and anger at being dominated. This is parallel to the excuses men give to justify hitting their wives, such as a woman's being unfaithful....In my opinion, [these] are not feminist critiques, but justifications of violence by women in the guise of feminism. This is the betrayal of the feminist ideal of a nonviolent world. In addition, excusing violence by women and denying overwhelming research evidence may have serious side effects. It may undermine the credibility of feminist scholarship and contribute to a backlash that can also undermine progress toward the goal of equality between men and women.[7]

Like Steinmetz, Straus believes that many of the arguments used against such research have the same tone that was used against the early research about wife battering. They remember well the dismissive arguments, as they were leaders in bringing wife abuse to the public's attention in the early 1970s. Straus holds out the hope that in the future we will wonder what today's argument is about.

The family violence study research is often assailed for including only assaults that happen during a marriage and not after a separation or divorce. Straus and his fellow researchers at the project have never tried to hide the fact that this is an area that is not part of their study; indeed, they consistently point it out. Other researchers have examined this question and found similar results.

The more recent National Violence Against Women Survey did ask questions about sexual assault and the questions were very specific, which is an area earlier research often neglected. It should be pointed out, though, that other types of questions that males might be more likely to state as having happened were left out. Specifically, physical attacks that include scalding or burning, and sexual assaults that include kicking or hitting in the groin.

R. L. McNeely is an attorney and a professor of social welfare at the University of Wisconsin at Milwaukee. In 1987, he wrote a paper for the journal of the National Association of Social Workers (*Social Work*) called "The Truth about Domestic Violence: A Falsely Framed Issue." The coauthor was Gloria Robinson-Simpson. The article generated the same kind of reaction that Steinmetz received from the publication of her article in *Victimology*. Following the *Social Work* article, the chancellor of the university received a letter from a women's group in Pennsylvania saying that the article was "hogwash," that they would do everything in their power to see that any federal funding McNeely received would be terminated, and that any federal funding he might apply for in the future would not be forthcoming. "I found that a bit amusing," McNeely says. "Not only was my work not funded by the federal government; I don't plan on applying for any federal funds." Another incident was less amusing:

> I was interviewed for a deanship at Michigan State University. Initially, every-thing went fine; people seemed to be quite excited at my application. When I got there, things had cooled off considerably. When I went for my interview with the vice chancellor, on his desk was a copy of this article. His major question to me was, "What is this about?" That told me that someone had felt it necessary to make sure that he had a copy of the article. I am sure they accompanied the article with a letter about whatever their political position was. Needless to say, I didn't really hear about a dean's position at that uni-versity after I left.[8]

McNeely says Robinson-Simpson's work on the paper was dismissed in some quarters as a woman who was under the domination of a male professor. He agrees with Steinmetz that the element of the feminist community that seeks to discredit the researchers on domestic violence who also mention vio-lence against men is a small, vocal minority:

> However, they are a very powerful minority. You have to realize that they are not about the search for truth. What this is about is a search for political power. That is power based upon a concept of a defenseless group of people being victimized by a larger, stronger aggressor. When people start recogniz-ing that, indeed, domestic violence seems to occur both ways, that under-cuts the whole concept of weakness, out of which comes power. It's based on a concept of being an exclusive victim. That's why some people react so strongly. A lot of these people are absolutely convinced that they are on the "correct" side. They are not going to listen to anything that undercuts that. But, it's not necessary for this information to do that [hurt the campaign against wife battering]. If we are really talking about reducing violence, we re not going to do it by talking about only one side of the problem. We have to confront it, no matter where it occurs. If people were to join together on that basis, then it would strengthen the effort against all types of domestic violence.

McNeely and Robinson-Simpson argue in their paper that the failure to recognize a significant portion of domestic violence negatively affects public policy:

> [It] is based on the assumption that men, exclusively or nearly exclusively, perpetrate domestic assaults. Thus, the public, legislators, change agents, and other activists are acting on underlying assumptions that may be false or at best, not fully reflective of domestic violence. Policies, then, are being

built on an erroneous vision of physical abuse. Accounts of domestic violence reinforce the dominant view by excluding any reference to the pervasiveness of violence in American families, and, almost invariably, by ignoring male victimization.[9]

ACADEMIC SUPPRESSION

While McNeely, Straus, and Steinmetz have been the subjects of somewhat well-known efforts to inhibit and suppress their work on male victimization, it is difficult to determine what other chilling effects might be taking place in the cloistered halls of academia. The continued absence of something is more difficult to prove than its presence.

It has not gone entirely unnoticed, however. Murray Straus and Donald Dutton are just two of the highly regarded and much-published researchers who have taken the time to investigate and point out a number of examples of published work that hides evidence of male abuse; avoids obtaining evidence or suppresses contrary evidence; practices selective citation; publishes conclusions that are not in the data; and denies funding to research that might contradict patriarchy oriented gender-feminist theory.

Here are but a few samples of this type:

Ask women only about victimization and ask men only about violence they perpetrate: Example: National Survey of Child and Adolescent Well-Being

If both victimization and perpetration questions are asked, publish only the data on male perpetration: Example: Johnson and Leone Study of "Intimate Terrorists" The Differential Effects of Intimate Terrorism and Situational Couple Violence—Findings from the National Violence Against Women Survey, *Journal of Family Issues,* 26 (3), 322–349.

Only men could be intimate terrorists because they did not analyze the data on violence by women.

Publish conclusions that are not in the data: Example: Poco Kernsmith, "Exerting Power or Striking Back: A Gendered Comparison of Motivations for Domestic Violence Perpetration," *Victims and Violence* 20 (2005): 173. "Males and females were found to differ in their motivations for using violence in relationships. Females reported using violence in response to prior abuse, citing revenge and retaliation as a primary motivation." This is an example of "finding" a gender difference when the data show none.

Deny funding to research that might contradict the patriarchy theory: Example: December 2005, National Institute of Justice call for proposals to investigate partner violence and sexual violence; it stated that studies of male victims are not eligible for funding.[10]

Besides academia, there have been other incidents of threatened violence against those who chose to publicly speak out on the issue of abused men.

I was part of a panel at a symposium in Vancouver, British Columbia, and the featured speaker was Canadian Senator Anne Cools. She was a pioneer in first introducing legislation and providing support for battered women in Canada. Perhaps that is why the protestors felt so threatened, but she was prevented from speaking by a group of 40 or so women who not only shouted down her every polite attempt to speak or even create a dialogue with them but also constantly blew loud police whistles. Eventually, they got so close to her that others and I were concerned about her physical safety. When one local TV station arrived to cover the incident, the protesters said that males in the audience had assaulted them. One man got irritated at the police whistle in his ear and grabbed it out of the protestor's hand. The reporter accepted that the protestor had been "assaulted" by a male without question. My own experience at one domestic violence conference (where I had received permission from organizers to hand out flyers about this book) was a bit scary when a very big man—I've met a couple of NFL linebackers and he was their size—approached me. He was ashamed enough about what he was doing to hide his name tag when he got right in my face, herded me into a corner, and loudly told me I wasn't welcome (I later found out that he is a physician).

There is concrete information about studies in which the data on assaults by women were intentionally suppressed. A survey conducted by the Kentucky Commission on Women in 1979, which was sponsored by the U.S. Department of Justice and the Law Enforcement Assistance Administration and was issued as a government report, failed to report the male victimization rates uncovered by the survey. The existence of the data became known only after other researchers obtained the computer tape and found that, among violent couples, 38 percent were attacks by women on men, who, as reported by the women themselves, had not been attacked by their male mates.[11]

A respected researcher at a university had a work on female murderers held hostage for a year. The initial draft was accepted by the university press with only minor corrections and suggestions noted. When it was submitted for final review, it was obvious that the first draft had been given to a wider variety of people beyond the initial review committee, and the final review committee makeup was changed. The new head of the review committee wanted major changes, which had to include studies of male murderers as "balance." Of course, that was not the focus of this researcher's book; had it been a study of both genders, it would have been constructed that way initially. The researcher was bound by contract to publish first in the university press and could not seek another publisher without permission. It took a long political fight, and uncommon tenacity, to finally get the work approved for release.

It would take another book to print all the examples of skewed data published by some in the academic community that have as their clear purpose an attempt to minimize female violence and downplay male victimization. To give yet another example, a paper published by the World Health Organization said that, "Where violence by women occurs, it is more likely to be in the form of self-defense."[12] A bold and sweeping claim, and the researchers duly cited references to back it up. When the references are examined, however, the claim falters: one did not even look at self-defense, the other survey showed the opposite—that it was not more likely to be self-defense when women do it, and the other references simply had no data at all. The paper also failed to cite at least nine other studies that found that the percentage of intimate partner violence that is self-defensive only in nature is about the same for men and women. There is widespread suspicion among many members of the academic community who study family violence issues that these examples are but a few among many.

I'll leave it up to the social scientists to debate whether this type of thing is more or less prevalent in this particular field compared to other social issues. There is, at least, more than a suspicion among many in the field that it is worse.

KILL THE MESSENGER

A primary criticism of the research that shows some women as well as some men to be violent in domestic relationships is that there is no context, that is, there is no differentiation among the acts noted. Some feminists argue that the results are skewed and therefore irrelevant, because the women may be acting in self-defense or as a result of provocation. The self-reporting by women of a significant number of initiated attacks in the general population surveys demonstrate, though, that the findings cannot be that easily dismissed.

If we accept this argument, what about the men who may be acting in self-defense? Data that come from women who have sought services at domestic violence shelters are biased and unrepresentative of the general population. It is interesting to note, however, that during the rare times such women are asked the question, the results show that a significant percentage of the women themselves state they have been violent.

In his incisive work *Not Guilty: The Case in Defense of Men,* David Thomas interviewed Erin Pizzey. We mentioned Pizzey in Chapter 1 as the author of *Scream Quietly, or the Neighbors Will Hear.* She is, to general acknowledgment, the founder of the movement to recognize domestic violence as a serious social issue. Her book was the first. She also set up the world's first shelter for battered women, Chiswick Women's Refuge, in London. Battered women owe her a great debt.

Like Straus and Steinmetz, though, Pizzey has been excommunicated from feminist ranks. How can this be? She dared to show that women, as well as men, can be violent. Indeed, her 1982 book *Prone to Violence* resulted in greater malevolence than that which greeted the work of Straus and Steinmetz. The publisher was threatened with having his windows smashed. Pizzey was picketed, and the London police insisted that she have an escort for her book tour in England. Someone shot at her home in the United States.

Her crime? She noted that a 1975 study of 100 women who visited the shelter found that 62 participated in a mutually violent relationship. She told Thomas that the women were both the victims and the perpetrators of regular acts of aggression. Some were more violent than the men they were seeking shelter from. Pizzey told Thomas:

> Time and again I've dealt with men who are physically attacked by women. In fact, the ophthalmologist I used to go to in Santa Fe [New Mexico] said that one of the major injuries he saw was men who had bottles and glasses in their eyes. I suppose that at the end of five years in America, in which I traveled and lectured everywhere from Alaska to the South, I just came to the conclusion that not only did I have hardly any American women friends, but they were the most aggressive and dangerous women I'd ever met in the world…terrifying.

Pizzey doubts the sincerity of many in the shelter movement. Hers is an interesting view in contrast to those who suspect that anyone speaking out against abuse directed at males is not so much interested in domestic violence as in a political agenda:

> I remember sitting in the offices of the women's movement in London, watching the activists come in, ripping open these letters from desperate women, putting the money in their pockets—because it cost three pounds, ten shillings to join—and then throwing the letters into the back of a cupboard. Many of the early refuges weren't really shelters for battered women and children—sure, they'd have a couple—but a means of getting grants.
>
> There are as many violent women as men, but there's a lot of money in hating men, particularly in the United States—millions of dollars. It isn't a politically good idea to threaten the huge budgets for women's refuges by saying that some of the women who go into them aren't total victims. Anyway, the activists aren't there to help women come to terms with what's happening in their lives. They're there to fund their budgets, their conferences, their traveling abroad, and their statements against men.[13]

The point here is not to excuse violence, no matter who started it or what the provocation was. True self-defense is another matter. Research shows, however, that in the overwhelming majority of domestic violence cases a direct threat to one's life is not involved. If we excuse the violent acts of women by saying that they must have been provoked, or were acting in response to violent acts by men, we would have to accept violent acts by men under the same circumstances.

This is a spurious and dangerous argument. It shows more of a concern for protecting an exclusive victim power base rather than a concern about domestic violence. Excusing violence by either sex endangers both women and men. Research shows that when one partner hits, the other partner is more likely to engage in violence. It perpetuates a view of the marriage license as a hitting license.

FACTS JUST GET IN THE WAY

Whereas critics of researchers like Straus and Steinmetz continually point to what they perceive as inaccuracies or, more often, failure to put the data in the context of male domination, the record is replete with enormous extrapolations and convoluted logic by many of these same detractors. There seems to be a tendency among some in the battered women's movement to overstate the case by using unscientific "evidence" in an effort to call attention to the seriousness of the problem. Why they should deem this necessary, when the factual evidence that does exist is bad enough, is not readily understood. It may be the result of simple overzealousness on behalf of a cause they feel passionate about. Whatever the reason, these kinds of statements tend to backfire and hurt the cause of reducing domestic violence against women and men.

It is not necessary to give a long list of examples in this regard; a few will do. It would serve no useful purpose to comb press reports and point out a substantial number of discrepancies that should have been checked, or at least questioned, by members of the news media. As a daily journalist for a number of years, I know too well that the greatest failure of journalism is not what *is* printed or broadcast but what is *not* printed or broadcast. Unlike what many members of the public may believe, this is for the most part not due to a desire to suppress information or skew the story toward a particular political ideology; rather, it can be attributed to simple laziness. It is much easier to accept seemingly "official" pronouncements as fact, and get the story out quickly, than to delve into the background of those "facts." Once a "statistic" gets accepted by one reporter, other reporters tend to accept it as well. These statements then can take on a life of their own and, regardless of the source, when repeated often enough become accepted as credible fact.

I appreciate the work of David Lees in his article in *Toronto Life:*

> The statistic that one disabled woman in two has been sexually assaulted at some point in her life carries a visceral charge—the damning implication that helplessness and vulnerability incite the sexual rage of men. [This statistic was given in support of domestic violence legislation in the Canadian

House of Commons by a member of Parliament.] The finding, which seems to show up more frequently than any other in the rhetoric of the women's movement, comes out of a 1986 study funded in part by the Ontario Ministry of Community and Social Services.[14]

Lees reports that this so-called fact was based on a questionnaire that was distributed at a conference of the Dis-Abled Women's Network (DAWN), an organization funded by the federal Women's Program. Thirty disabled women filled out the questionnaire. This self-selected group, who had all expressed an advance interest in the issue, could by no means be a representative sample of all disabled women.

Lees says Member of Parliament Edna Anderson took the questionnaire results and claimed in the House of Commons that 40 percent of disabled women had been sexually or physically assaulted as adults. This statement, a twisting of data to fit a political agenda, was based on 18 of the women saying they had not been assaulted, 5 not answering the question, and 7 saying they had been assaulted. Anderson apparently got to 40 percent by adding the 5 women who didn't answer the questionnaire one way or the other with the 7 who said they were assaulted.

This questionnaire has also been used to claim that almost 50 percent of disabled women were sexually assaulted as children. Left out of this statement is who did the assaulting, even according to the flawed survey. Fourteen women said they had been the victims of childhood sexual abuse. Of the 14, 2 were assaulted by women—by a mother and a female relative. The same group, when asked about physical abuse as children, revealed that in 8 cases the batterers were mothers, fathers battered in 6 instances, and female caregivers battered in 5 cases. Lees says that Anderson and others blithely reporting "results" from a flawed study seem to be less concerned with the plight of disabled women and more concerned with making a case against men and portraying them as sexual abusers.

This Canadian case history of a "fact" with a life of its own and its uncritical acceptance by the news media is not unique to Canada or to this one instance. In an excerpt from her book *Who Stole Feminism?*—reported in the *National Review*—writer Christina Hoff Sommers examined another fact with a life of its own. In this case, though the information was fabricated, it found uncritical acceptance. In 1992, Deborah Louis, president of the National Women's Studies Association, informed members through an electronic bulletin board that the March of Dimes reported that domestic violence against pregnant women causes more birth defects than all other causes combined. This information was then given out by the San Francisco Family Violence Prevention Fund and by Sarah Buel of the Domestic Violence Advocacy Project at Harvard

Law School. The *Boston Globe, Dallas Morning News,* and *Time* magazine, among other media outlets, all dutifully reported that a March of Dimes study said that battering of women during pregnancy is the leading cause of child birth defects. *Time* later printed a correction when it found out that the March of Dimes had never issued such a report.[15]

It turns out that Buel had misunderstood a statement by a child care specialist with the March of Dimes, who had said that more women are screened for birth defects than are screened for domestic battery. That's quite a different statement from domestic violence being the *cause* of more birth defects than all other causes. While the *Time* correction had already appeared, and the March of Dimes media relations office was busy denying the existence of such a report to other members of the media as well as to officials who were calling, Buel was apparently unaware of her error. Sommers reports that when she informed her of the error, Buel was about to use this "fact" in yet another article.

Reporter Joe Hallinan of the Newhouse News Service examined another so-called fact that gained widespread uncritical acceptance in the news media: the statement that domestic violence is the leading cause of injury to women between the ages of 15 and 44. Or sometimes, more simply, the leading cause of injury to women. On the face of it, such a statement would seem highly improbable. More women injured by domestic violence than by car accidents and accidents in the home? Surely, some journalists would want to question the primary source directly on such a broad and unlikely statement. Hallinan found out that a long list of respectable news organizations reported it, including *Time, Newsweek, the Washington Post,* CNN, ABC, and others.

Hallinan did some checking. The news organizations (pointed in this direction by advocacy groups) cited a letter by former Surgeon General Antonia Novello printed in the *Journal of the American Medical Association* (*JAMA*) as their source. Novello gave as her source a Philadelphia study done by a University of Pennsylvania professor. When Hallinan questioned this researcher, the professor pointed out that the study was concentrated almost entirely on poor inner-city black women and should by no means be used to represent the entire population of women. Second, even in this study, there was not a distinction between domestic violence–caused injuries and injuries caused by strangers. Apparently, Novello never actually made the claim of more injuries due to domestic violence among women. The Domestic Violence and Injury Survey in the Appendix has the full report of the University of Pennsylvania study.

Hallinan found that numerous politicians and members of the press have also reported that domestic violence not only is the most common cause of injury to women, it is more common than cancer, heart attacks, rape, muggings, or even all of these combined. The cancer comment source? Novello again, who said it in a speech after the letter in *JAMA*. A colleague who co-wrote the letter told Hallinan than Novello apparently misspoke when she made the cancer comment in the speech; there is no study backing this claim. As for domestic violence being a more common cause of injury to women than heart attacks, rape, muggings, or car accidents, muggings, and rapes combined, the beginning source (1985) is apparently Evan Stark and Anne Flitcraft of Connecticut, with the approval of frequent reprints of the statement in the *Journal of the American Medical Association* and in the popular news media. They examined hospital emergency room medical records of women who reported injuries and compared them with the number of auto accidents, muggings, and rapes. They apparently classified *any* injury caused by another person (stranger or not) as a possible case of domestic violence. Stark told Hallinan that the medical record usually noted when the injury was caused by a stranger; if there was no notation, they *assumed* it was a case of domestic violence. They classified the injury total into four types: positive, probable, suggestive, or negative. They apparently combined the positive, probable, and suggestive types to reach a total that was greater than the other combined causes of injury. When interviewed by Hallinan, however, Stark admitted that even their conclusions cannot be taken to mean that domestic violence is the leading cause of injury since there may be other forms of injury that have not been examined. He agreed that the best that could be said about the study is that "maybe domestic violence is the leading cause of injury and maybe it isn't."[16]

Following the first edition of this book, I undertook a project to explore just how widely this one erroneous *factoid* was repeated by those in authority. I had to give up after I found more than 100 organizations and prominent individuals who had made this claim. Mostly, I did not even bother to look at organizations that had as their purpose service or advocacy for domestic violence victims. The complete list compiled is in the Appendix. The list runs from a president to senators, and organizations like the American College of Surgeons and the Brain Injury Institute, and many other established organizations and prominent individuals, such as district attorney offices, law enforcement agencies, and public health care organizations. I also include a detailed critique of other false and/or misleading statements by the American College of Surgeons' Web site at the time of the survey.

Frankly, I was astonished. Yet, it reflects and supports the view that there is more false, falsely framed, or disingenuously deceptive information about domestic violence than any other significant public and social issue.

How could, for example, the U.S. Department of Health and Human Services for eight long years put on its Web site the claim that "Domestic violence is the leading cause of injury to women"? Surely, a first-year medical student would question that claim—greater than household accidents?

It took two years, letters from a congressman, and an inquiry from a senator's office, plus numerous letters, which mostly went unanswered, for an undersecretary at HHS to finally respond that maybe "the" leading cause was erroneous, but it was "a" leading cause. The truth, of course, is that it is neither. Eventually, HHS removed the statement from its Web site but refused to issue a retraction, even after eight years of perpetrating an outrageously false "health" statement.

Former Secretary of Health and Human Services Donna Shalala also told the American Medical Association's National Conference on Family Violence that, "We do know that 20 to 30 percent of the injuries that send women to the emergency room stem from physical abuse by their partners."[17]

Even if we assume that all of the unknown relationship assaults in the Justice Department ER survey were due to domestic violence, that still would not approach 30 percent of all ER admissions for women, or even 20 percent.

The Centers for Disease Control, in its "National Hospital Ambulatory Medical Care Survey: 1992 Emergency Department Summary," shows that the leading cause of injury, to both women and men, is accidental falls, followed by motor vehicle accidents. According to the CDC, 13.6 percent of injuries to women seen in emergency rooms are from car accidents—a total of nearly 2 million, or almost 10 times the number of injuries from domestic violence. Twice as many women visit emergency rooms due to being injured by an animal (459,000 a year) than by a male partner.

In addition, the most recent U.S. Justice Department Survey (NCJ-156921) of injury-related visits to emergency rooms found that *all* violence is responsible for 3 percent of such visits and domestic violence for 1 percent. In total, this means that domestic violence accounts for fewer than 0.3 percent of ER visits. Despite careful charting procedures, it is true that the relationship to the assailant was unknown for one-fifth of the female patients and fully one-third of the male assault violence victims who represented 14 percent and 3 percent, respectively, of all intimate partner assault victims in the national sample (79 hospital) survey. Even if, however, the assumption is made that all of the unknown relationship assault victims were included as domestic violence, it still would not even be close to true that domestic violence is *a* leading cause, and certainly not *the* leading cause, of injury to women (or men) at any age.[18]

"Every 12 seconds another woman is beaten. That's nearly 900,000 victims every year." When President Clinton made this statement, his math was off. Nine hundred thousand victims a year does not equal one every 12 seconds, but what's really eyebrow-raising is that the figure of 900,000 is closer to the number of *male* victims each year. Clinton was noting in his address to the nation the signing into law of the reauthorization of the Violence Against Women Act (nearly $5 billion over five years). That survey found 1.5 million female victims each year, and 835,000 male victims.[19]

It is not the position of this book to downplay the injuries caused by domestic violence to women or to men. It is important, however, to serve up a note of caution. Simply because sources seem to be authoritative doesn't mean the methods used to determine the results shouldn't be carefully examined.

The urban myth about greater domestic violence occurring on Super Bowl Sunday still has its repeaters among the news media on this day each year, despite the fact that those who first put the story out had to admit that there was no accurate survey available that shows it is true, even among shelter providers. The idea is widespread that men in the military "must" be more violent toward their mates than men in other professions, although there is no evidence to support this contention (as demonstrated in Chapter 1). These are just two examples of the myths and unexamined claims that gain acceptance because they seem to fit current common conceptions, seem to come from authoritative sources, and are not subject to adequate journalistic scrutiny or critical thinking and examination.

The failure of adequate scrutiny means that a green light is given to those who play fast and loose with unqualified and perspective-less facts in promotion of an emotional cause at the expense of an objective view. There does seem to be a pattern that those who engage in this activity as opposed to those activists who speak more carefully are the very same persons who can be relied upon to downplay, minimize, and protest against any recognition that men can be victims of domestic violence.

NEWS MEDIA BIAS

The news media, unfortunately, can be sexist. It is often the case that when a domestic violence story in which a man is the victim draws the popular press attention, it is treated as a general crime story and the words *domestic violence* or *spouse abuse* are not used. The story of Steven Moskowitz, detailed in Chapter 2, is one example of this different kind of treatment. The murder of comedian Phil Hartman at the hands of his wife is but one further example. Indeed, the list of male celebrities who have in court documents accused their wives and girlfriends of assaults, or police reports have confirmed, is quite long, and range from professional football players to prominent actors and singers. Humphrey Bogart? Kelsey Grammer? The list of female celebrity victims covered by the news media or in court/police records is even longer, as compiled by several domestic violence awareness organizations. My Web site www. abusedmen.com will likely contain such a list.

It is not our purpose here to play a male/female celebrity numbers game, but to examine how the news media reacts and reports on such items. Celebrity cases naturally attract more media attention than do things that happen to others. It seems to me that the news media in general has not changed much in the past 10 years in this respect, that a fair assessment of such stories finds a general lack of the words *domestic violence* when associated with male victims, celebrity or not. When such an incident happens in a dramatic enough way to attract news media attention or even in a much smaller general crime section of a local newspaper, there has only been some small improvement in terms of using the words *domestic violence* and associating it with male victims as they most commonly do for female victims. Because editors and publishers and policies change, and this second edition will likely remain in print for a long time, I do not want to mention the name here, but it is notable that at least one daily medium-sized newspaper in New Jersey has adopted a stated policy that male and female victims of domestic violence will be covered in an equal manner and the words *domestic violence* will be used regardless of the gender of the victim. This newspaper is to be commended, but as near as can be determined, it is the only daily newspaper in the United States that has adopted a formal policy in this regard.

Sometimes when a man is the victim, there is even an attempt to treat the story humorously.

John Griffith is a correspondent for *The Oregonian,* the state's largest daily newspaper. He wrote what he calls a fairly straightforward account of a woman who attacked her husband with a tire iron on their honeymoon. The husband suffered a severe concussion and broken fingers. At the editor's desk, Griffith's lead was changed, and this headline was added: "Husband Survives the Lumps and Bumps of a New Marriage." The lead paragraph read as follows: "Authorities aren't saying much, but one thing is clear: The recent marriage of a South Carolina couple who have been honeymooning on the Oregon coast has proved bumpy. Most of the bumps are on the husband's head."[20]

Griffith agrees that the lead is an attempt to be humorous. He says, "If it had been a woman who was injured, it probably would not have been treated that way. Any sort of lighthearted treatment would be viewed as grossly politically incorrect. If it had been a woman attacked, and it was written that way, people would have been aghast. You can imagine the heat they would have taken on that. It would have inspired a lot of negative comment."

Griffith says the paper received only one letter of protest. The wife who tried to kill her husband eventually received five years in prison. The prosecution proved she tried to kill her husband for a $1.4 million insurance policy.[21]

In England, Malcolm George says his research on male victims has resulted in numerous broadcast and print reports. By and large, he says they have been balanced reports and he has been fairly quoted; however, he notes an interesting phenomena:

> There have been fifty or sixty female reporters who have interviewed me, but as I pointed out to a BBC reporter, there have been only four male reporters. I can only speculate why this is so, but I think the answer is fairly obvious.

The male reporters are afraid they will be accused of sexist bias, if they do the reporting. Beyond that, there is the visceral response which may not be even realized. The whole subject makes men uncomfortable, perhaps even more so than women.[22]

That is an interesting interpretation, but then at least in television news, there are more female reporters than male ones, so George's take could be merely an effect of the news media population.

If male journalists find themselves inhibited from reporting on this topic, this may partially explain why there had been so little news media or other media coverage of the phenomenon in the past and even at the present day. Female reporters may also be inhibited from paying attention to the reality of male spousal abuse because it may result in a negative reaction from some feminists, within and outside of the newsroom. Retired CBS TV anchor Walter Cronkite has pointed out that it takes courage to be a journalist, a kind of courage that he sees in increasingly short supply in the profession—"not the courage to face bullets covering a war but the courage to face the dismay and disapproval of the public and particularly one's boss, colleagues, and friends in bringing to the public's attention an important but controversial topic." If Cronkite is correct in his assessment, certainly the subject of abused men currently qualifies as an issue that some journalists may lack the inclination or courage to pursue.[23]

Then, there is outright unthinking sexism (which affects both female and male reporters), not only in general terms of how men and women are "supposed" to be, but in more subtle ways as well, that sometimes is not even recognized as sexist behavior.

For example, I was contacted by a producer for the Oprah Winfrey show to do the topic. It was the first time apparently that this show had ever covered the issue. It was a very well-done show in my opinion, and I note that this show has conducted several subsequent shows on the topic. Though I was the first person to be contacted about the topic, I put them in touch with many others, suggested male victims who would appear, and so on; this included a female therapist who works primarily with female perpetrators, not male victims. She did a good job and I have no qualms about it and am always grateful when public discourse on the issue is promoted. The sexism came into play when the producer told me why I was not selected to be the "expert guest." I was male. They wanted "balance" on the topic. The producers have had no qualms about a female speaking on behalf of female victims on previous shows about domestic violence. In other words, women can be advocates for both female and male victims, but males cannot be public advocates for male victims.

A 10-YEAR SEA CHANGE

Has there been an increase in news media coverage of male victims since *Abused Men* was first published? If so, has there been an effect on increasing public recognition in general, and most important, in the provision of services?

A 100 percent increase sounds impressive, but if the increase represents going from zero to one, the total numbers do not add up to much. One must be cautious. Since the first edition, however, my circle of acquaintances has increased. Additionally, there are now at least six nationally intent organizations (two public policy focused rather than nonprofit service oriented) concerned with increasing recognition for abused men. They did not exist 10 years ago. As might be expected, they have reported most of their news media "successes" to me, and even ones that did not originate due to their input. Then, there are those members of the news media that have contacted me directly. Suffice it to say, I probably am best qualified to answer these two questions.

The Media

Except for the Hallinan Newhouse Newspapers story noted earlier and in the first edition, this was the only national outlet I could find at the time that devoted any coverage to the general issues involved. Today, *60 minutes* (CBS network) and *Dateline* (NBC-MSNBC has covered the topic once) are the holdouts in failing to make an *inquiry* at least about a possible story; most have done full segments or covered related news items and mentioned fairly accurate current statistics. The majority of U.S. nationally broadcast news media have covered the issue, some more than once (*20/20, O'Reilly Factor*). Besides the hard news–oriented shows (except the specifically politics-only shows), this would include all of the entertainment talk shows such as *Montel Williams* (except *The View*)., and even so-called light entertainment and information national television shows such as the *Home and Family Network* (now defunct). The network morning shows (except for CNN and MSNBC), however, have yet to do the topic, although they have all made inquiries. Some 20 local television news outlets have done stories, including an extraordinary by local TV news standards half-hour mini-doc by the Washington, DC, Fox News station.

At least two nationally broadcast radio talk shows have covered the issue, as have about 50 local radio talk shows, and the number of local daily newspapers, as well as college newspapers, that have covered the topic is about the same. Both the Canadian and U.S. national Associated Press wire have printed stories on the subject. Copyright issues prevent me from printing the entire U.S. A.P. wire feature article in the Appendix, but I thought it was particularly fair and the national reporter talked with an equal number of critics of recognition as well as supporters; most of these comments in the A.P. national features story (which means it appeared in many daily newspapers across the United States) appeared in Chapter 1. I also am aware of articles in daily newspapers (in the UK, Australia, and Canada—some national), and quite a number of these, particularly UK, daily newspapers have covered the issue more than once.

Two nationally syndicated advise columnists (Dear Abby and Ask Amy) have featured the issue in their columns. There is news also on the issue out of India and Taiwan, more than other places it seems, and a little bit out of Japan. Not being fluent in other languages except for Spanish, it is more difficult for me to assess any increases in coverage in other countries. From what I can determine, there appears to be an increase in coverage in Germany and France.

I expect there to be continued news media coverage over the next 10 years at about the same steady pace. Some conclude that they have done the story once, so there is not a need to do it again, despite the fact that there are many related current issues beyond the simple one that there is proof that men are being abused by their female mates. Unless, of course, there is that celebrity or particularly notorious nationally covered incident that always excites the news media, and that may further increase media attention.

On the other hand, the politics of the issue have been totally ignored by the news media and all political parties. The U.S. Violence Against Women Act and its equivalent in Canada and other countries attract a large amount of tax dollars. In the United States, it amounts to an average of $1 billion a year. That's not small change even by Washington, DC, standards. I'll have more on VAWA and some of the changes in the law itself in the concluding chapter, and the Appendix has a list of current problems in the law. Unfortunately, the Appendix report points out problems in the law, but says little about remedies. It seems that there would be at least some media attention and even political or policy debate surrounding this much funding, but it has been entirely lacking.

Services

Has there been an increase in services for male victims in the past 10 years? What are the prospects for a steady growth in services in the future?

The increase in actual shelter services is demonstrable, as verified by the Washington, DC, television station; there was only one shelter in the United States that also served men (the Valley Oasis shelter in the desert of Lancaster, California) 10 years ago. Unfortunately, it is impossible to say with certitude just how many there actually are today. There is now one national toll-free hotline (DAHMW) that does not discriminate against men and endeavors to find real resources for them—carefully checking out each referral to a local service organization—but it is not the vastly more recognized and well-funded

National Domestic Violence Hotline from the National Coalition Against Domestic Violence. A non–toll-free hotline also exists (SAFE, Stop Abuse For Everyone). We just don't know how many hotlines there are. It would be safe to say, however, that there are at least half a dozen and perhaps as many as a dozen in the United States.

There were just a few crisis lines that didn't discriminate 10 years ago, now there are many more. How many, we can't say for sure, and organizations go through change. However, a note of caution is needed. Some crisis lines make a public statement that they serve men, but when tested by actual male callers, they sometimes do not.

A southern Florida shelter and crisis line I know of, for example, declares that it serves men, but a former worker at the shelter told me that in reality, it does not. The National Coalition of Free Men carried out an extensive test in Los Angeles. They had a male call 10 shelters in the area. All 10 denied services; none would even give him a hotel arrangement or other shelter services.

It is interesting to note, however, that I was at one of the nation's largest domestic violence conferences in San Diego and the moderator of a well-attended (300 or so) break-out session asked the audience how many of them now served abused men as well as women. The moderator guessed that about one-third of the audience raised their hands. I don't think that 10 years ago that many would have raised their hands at a domestic violence conference, and indeed, the question would never have been asked.

On the other hand, while that was a positive gain for recognition and per-haps an indicator of increased services, it is instructive to note how nervous those in the established domestic violence movement are to even the men-tion of the existence of abused men. I gave a break-out session talk at this same convention, but the organizer of the conference felt compelled to take me aside and warn me against being too controversial—simply because of the mere mention of abused men as a topic open for discussion. The organizers also (at the last minute and in violation of their earlier agreement) decided to add—thereby cutting my time in half—the presentation of a young woman who simply told her personal story of being the victim of abuse, even though the title of the seminar was "Abused Men."

In a much smaller venue (a local domestic violence coordinating commit-tee composed of judges, probation officers, law enforcement agents, shelter and crisis line representatives, and other providers of services), the issue of greater recognition and services for male victims came up. The steady gaze of one female police officer who told an objector to this policy that it was the law that they not practice sexual discrimination struck me in a forceful way. It must have struck the objector as well—the vote for inclusion of an organiza-tion that supported such a policy was successful.

At another conference on gay, lesbian, bisexual, and transgendered victims of domestic violence, there were statements made about violent women by female speakers that would most likely not have been allowed to be said 10 years ago.

On the other hand, when it comes to the true nature of domestic violence in all its aspects, by many domestic violence service providers, there is much to be discouraged about. At another conference, the speaker was talking about the recidivism rate of male perpetrators. A valid topic to be sure, but I mentioned to my tablemate that maybe the recidivism rate of victims needs to be addressed as well. That is, people who return again and again to the same or same type of violent relationship. He told me, "You'd better not mention that word and victims in the same breath around here." The drumbeat at the majority of domestic violence conferences remains solely focused on female victims and while it may be the reality faced by these providers, examining patterns of behavior by women in these situations is forbidden and any talk of the predominate paradigm of mutual combat or how best to deal with it is not on the table.

PUBLIC ATTITUDES

Unfortunately, we have only one test of public attitudes about intimate partner violence that examines gender differences. A new study has not been conducted since 1992. Two questions were asked:

1. "Are there any situations that you can imagine in which you would approve of a husband slapping his wife's face?"
2. "Are there any situations that you can imagine in which you would approve of a wife slapping her husband's face?"

The preliminary results show that approval of slapping by husbands decreased from a high of 20 percent in 1968, to 13 percent in 1985, and 12 percent in 1992. However, approval of slapping by wives remained unchanged. It was 22 percent in 1968, 21.3 percent in 1985, and 22 percent in 1992. The results are demonstrated in graphic form in Figure 4.1. In general, fewer women than men approve of marital violence. However, the gender gap is narrowing because approval by men has decreased dramatically, whereas approval by women has decreased less or, in the case of slapping by women, has increased slightly. The researchers concluded:

> We suggest that one of the reasons for the large decrease in approval of slapping a wife reflects the efforts of the feminist movement to end male violence. Similarly, the fact that approval of slapping a husband has not decreased may reflect the absence of an equivalent campaign (and ameliorating programs) to end violence by women.[24]

Figure 4.1
Approval of Slapping a Spouse, 1968–1992

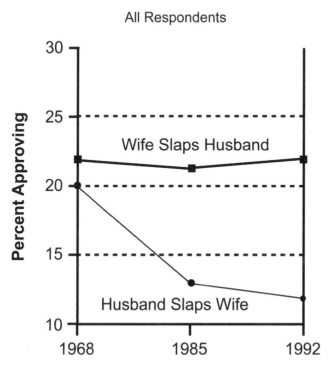

Courtesy of Murray A. Straus.

THE VIEW FROM HOLLYWOOD

There does seem to be some change occurring, both in attitude and awareness. Some popular books have been published with chapters on the subject of male domestic violence (Warren Farrell's *The Myth of Male Power* may be the most widely known), and the impact of the 1993 CBS TV movie *Men Don't Tell*, which was a fictionalized account of an abused husband, was extraordinary. The number of academically oriented books on the subject has increased (e.g., *The Whole Truth about Domestic Violence* by James Kline, Ph.D., a particularly fine review and critique of the literature and movement), and certainly there are a number of other books of more recent vintage touching on the particular subject of abused men (see Selected Bibliography). On the whole, however, it would be presumptuous to declare that there has been a large increase in books dealing with the subject in recent years.

Nancy Bein is the producer of the movie. She worked for CBS for nine years as the vice president for television movies and has some 400 TV movies to her credit. She has produced four movies as an independent producer since leaving the network. It seems extraordinary, but Bein insisted in the interview for this book that out of all those hundreds of movies, there is no doubt that the reaction to *Men Don't Tell* was the greatest:

> I find it incredible, with all the subjects that have been covered, that this was the first movie and that you're writing the first book. I decided to do this movie because a friend, who is a psychologist, told me about a client who was a police officer and who had been a victim of domestic violence. He told my friend that he always expected that each incident would be the last time, that he didn't hit her back because he was afraid he would really hurt her. She told my friend that she hit him to get his attention.
>
> So that's what started the whole idea, that there was this kind of syndrome happening out there. From the research that we did find, and there wasn't very much, we learned that it is very similar to what happens to battered women. First, that there generally has to be a history of physical or verbal abuse in the families of both perpetrator and victim; otherwise, it's not accepted. Secondly, it is almost like there is a nonverbal contract between the two, that this type of thing is going to be how they deal with their lives.

So you did the research, but how did you approach the script?

> We made a very conscious effort to make sure the man was very masculine, because a number of people when they heard about the subject felt that the man must be very wimpy. We actually made him blue-collar, being in a field where he was somewhat physical. Some of the writers that I had approached were horrified. I had contacted a team of two women writers who were very good. Both of them worked in a battered women's shelter, and they were incredibly offended. They tried to talk me out of doing it. Somehow they felt that any publicity about men being victims would somehow hurt the cause of women being victims, which I find very strange. It was a humanist film, in that nobody should be a victim. One of the writers who did work on the film, it turns out, told me afterward that they were the victim of family violence in that their mother went after their father. This writer gave us two of the wonderful scenes in the movie that were from real life. One is when the police were called by the neighbors and absolutely assumed that it was the husband battering the wife, as opposed to the way it was. The other is the scene where both of them go through the window. The father happened to be standing in a place where the mother came at him, and the way he moved, they both ended up crashing through the window. When we had completed the script, we began to make offers to stars. Judith Light said yes immediately. Peter Strauss was our second choice. Our first choice was an actor who said he was very offended that we sent him the script. He was angry at his agent for soliciting the script and forwarding it to him for him to read. Peter Strauss, a very bright man, accepted and did a very good job.

CBS was very high on the movie. They saw it as very high concept because it was one movie that hadn't been done before. They turned out to be right, as it did very well. It did very well overseas as well. It was one of the highest-rated movies of the year. Out of some 300 two-hour movies, I think it was rated number four, so it did extremely well. A lot of the reaction was that people turned it on with the idea of just to watch a few minutes but ended up being compelled to watch the whole movie and feeling very differently by the time it was finished.

What kind of reaction did you get?

I don't know what kind of response CBS got. The network is very compartmentalized, so what kind of letters and phone calls they got, I don't know.

I got a lot of letters directly sent to me, which surprised me. That's a hard thing to do. I was no longer at Lorimar [the production company that handled the movie]. I was at a different production company. The fact that people went to the trouble to get my name, spell it properly, call Lorimar, and track me down surprised me. Some letters went just to Lorimar. I also got a lot of phone calls, which is also a hard thing to do. Almost all of the letters and phone calls were from men. I found it remarkable that in all cases except one, every man left his first and his last name, either on the message slip or on the machine. It's part of the syndrome; "men don't tell" that they are ashamed. After the first couple of calls, it finally hit me why they were all doing that.

I think they were saying that it was not something to be ashamed of. This was one of the things that the movie emphasized, that you were not less of a man, or less of a human being, because this had happened to you. Yes, it was a problem, but dealing with it and recognizing it were actually very brave and courageous things to do. They wanted to volunteer, or learn about groups in their area. The man who wouldn't give his name was calling from a phone booth and stayed on hold a long time to wait for me. He wanted to know what he should do as a victim of violence, if he left, since he was being threatened with being killed. He wanted to know how to handle that situation. I told him to get in touch with a shelter. He was really frightened.

I got a call from a man in Florida who said that one incident which was shown in the movie happened to him. This was where the wife began to beat the husband when he was asleep. This man said that had happened to him, except that his wife beat him with a frying pan. Which we would never have dreamed of doing; it would be too over the top. This man was married for twenty-two years. He finally left. He got on a plane with just the money in his pocket, no job, and went to California. He slept on his sister's couch for months. He finally got a job and established himself. He had two sons. One is now married, and this son is now being battered by *his* wife. He wasn't sure what to do about it.

I got a letter from a woman who was a counselor at a battered woman's shelter. She was very angry initially that the movie was going to be aired. She wound up watching the whole movie and being very affected by it. She remembered men in groups who had brought up to her in the group or privately that they had been victims of violence, too. She had laughed at them. She had been very condescending. She felt horrible after seeing the movie. She went to her shelter and in a staff meeting talked about how important the movie was, and how it changed her perception, and that no one should be a victim. She said the staff treated her the same way that she treated those men. They derided her and thought that she was totally wrong. She said she understood for the first time how those men must feel. [Note: Steinmetz and I have received similar letters from counselors at shelters.]

Another letter was from a man who explained that both he and his girl-friend were victims of family violence while growing up. They each had terrible lives before they met each other, and each was nicer to the other than anybody had ever been in their entire lives. When she occasionally went off and battered him, he was furious. At the same time, he understood why she did it because he understood her family background. He loved her, and cared for her, and it didn't happen much, so he stayed.

It's an amazing [phenomenon] when someone sits down and writes you a two-page letter that is really heartfelt. That someone would take the time and energy to write to a stranger, that was a remarkable letter, but a lot of them were remarkable.

What did you tell these people? What advice did you give them?

Most didn't ask for advice. They wrote or called to tell their story and say thank you. They wanted me to know how important it was to do this movie. Some mentioned how they were going to call shelters and volunteer.

What kind of reaction did you get from those in the shelter movement?

All the ones that were negative initially had a very positive response after the movie. There were a number of shelters and groups that didn't say they were negative before it aired, didn't say either way, but now wanted a copy of the movie.[25]

A copy of the movie is not available for public sale. It was shown many times on Lifetime Cable TV, and was featured on the syndicated talk show *Sally Jesse Raphael,* which aired a program devoted to the movie and the general subject of domestic violence, and this same show also interviewed me and several male victims on a subsequent program.

Judith Light is the Emmy award-winning actress who played the abusing wife in the movie. Light has starred in a number of TV movies, as well as in series such as *Who's the Boss*. In an interview, I asked her whether she had some worries about accepting such a controversial role:

> At first I was really hesitant. I was extremely concerned that this issue would in some way taint the issue of men's abuse of women. I was not interested in doing anything that would take away from that issue.
>
> However, I was able to see the statistics that the producers showed us, and the information about how large a problem this was. I knew the producers, so I knew it would be well done. I knew that CBS would not be doing it unless it was important. What I wanted to do was expand the discussion of abuse across the board, as another form of abuse. As human beings, we are not restricted to one thing....The reaction was *extraordinary*. When you're making a movie, people commonly stop and ask the security person what it's about. People said to them, "Oh, yeah, that happens all the time." They didn't seem surprised. People on the set, in the crew, and so forth, came up to me and said, "Listen, you're telling my story." People came out of the closet like crazy. When I did the *Arsenio Hall Show* [just prior to the movie being aired], he asked for a show of hands on how many people in the audience knew of somebody who this has happened to, that a husband was abused by a wife. I would say a third to a half of the audience raised their hands.
>
> I got letters; I got calls. The network got calls. However, we couldn't put an 800 number on at the end of the movie because one doesn't exist. There's no place for men to go. They were calling CBS wanting to know how to get help, who to contact, what to do. There wasn't much CBS could tell them, except to tell them to talk to a counselor or mental health agency.
>
> I think men, just as women, need a place to go to feel safe and unburden themselves. We are all human beings. Everyone needs a place to feel safe. That doesn't make women bad, and it doesn't make men bad. It's just that both men and women have this problem on a psychological, physical, and spiritual level, that we all have to handle when it presents itself.[26]

Although a Canadian production company has produced a DVD about male abuse, the intent is primarily to educate those who work in shelters and crisis lines and is not the type of production the general public would be very interested in. Nancy Bein told me that she sees no reason why several popular consumption movies could not be produced about the subject, as many such movies have been made about abused women. Although *Disclosure* and *Fatal Attraction,* for example, do deal with stalking behavior by women against men, and there have been a few *Law and Order* episodes, Hollywood in the main has ignored the subject.

SILENT COUNSELORS

Because CBS had no place other than mental health agencies and private counselors to refer people to when they called for help at the time (and, unfortunately, due to lack of funding for publicity and media contact work, it probably would not even be aware today of organizations like the Domestic Abuse Hotline for Men and Women or Stop Abuse For Everyone), it is worth examining in further detail (beyond the comments of Sherven and Sniechowski in Chapter 3) how therapists and counselors respond to the abused male. In the main, the answer is simple: There is no response at all.

Seattle, Washington, area therapist Michael Thomas says the response of the therapeutic community is one of denial in that it is similar to the response of therapists and psychiatrists to abused women in the 1950s and 1960s: "It's all in your head. You've got a good husband. Here's some tranquilizers; now go home and try to make it better." While this may be an exaggeration, it was not an atypical response. Things have changed for the better in terms of response to abused women, but Thomas sees a parallel in the kinds of reaction and help women used to receive to what happens to abused men when they seek counseling:

> Today, I think there's very little minimizing for women who present as an abuse victim. If anything, there's almost a hyper-reaction. There's a great deal of minimizing of women's violence against men, by therapists, by the general community, by men themselves, and by women.
>
> In talking with other therapists, I find that they rarely even ask questions of their male clients about the possibility of the client being abused. It would be the rare clinician who would ask those kinds of questions, or even see what has happened to [the men] as being abusive or as serious. I think a great many clinicians are still resistant to seeing certain types of female behavior as abusive. If it does occur it is seen in terms of "no big deal" or "what did the man do to cause it?"
>
> If the client can't talk about it, it becomes internalized, and it increases the danger of the man exploding in rage himself, getting depressed or suicidal, withdrawing from relationships, and other kinds of possible effects. I have also heard from female abusers who can't get help. They call around and find that there are programs for male batterers and female victims, say, at a community health center, but not for the other side of the coin. If they do talk to a therapist, unfortunately, the frequent reaction is that they don't even see the possibility that the female can be a batterer. They say, "You're probably just fighting back, and you're the victim, and you just need to leave that relationship with an abusive man." There's very few resources out there, for either victim or abuser.[27]

Malcolm George in Great Britain says the same conditions exist there. He notes that one director of a domestic violence unit in England has discovered that there are a number of male victims, but she gets very few referrals from therapists or other mental health agencies. She also gets very few calls from the male victims themselves; usually, she is called by a relative or a second wife.

As we discovered, shame is a primary feeling among most male and female victims. If Thomas is right, that it is the rare therapist who even asks a man about his being abused, and it's only the occasional victim who is going to even mention it, then therapists will never know about a core problem for the client they are supposed to be helping.

No survey exists of therapists to see if attitudes have changed in this regard over the last 10 years. I suspect that there has been some improvement, but it is likely minimal.

On the other hand, there now exist nationally available user-friendly brochures (from SAFE) for male, gay, and lesbian victims of domestic violence. Therapists, hospitals, helping agencies, and law enforcement agencies have ordered more than 10,000 of these brochures.

GENDER-NEUTRAL LANGUAGE

The Portland, Oregon, area county corrections department has adopted the Duluth, Minnesota, Deferred Sentencing Program for domestic violence offenders, which is considered a national model. Chapter 5 will discuss details of this program and what it does. Despite the desire to be up to date with current thinking and approaches, however, the Portland program is typical of what is going on in similar domestic violence efforts around the United States: There is blatant and unapologetic sex discrimination.

In all the literature handed out to victims and perpetrators, as well as to the news media and to the public, gender-neutral language is forbidden. The perpetrator is always described as *he*. The victim is always *her*. Mark Hess, a coordinator with the Deferred Sentencing Program and one of the people on the front line in dealing with domestic violence offenders and victims, says:

> I don't think the language should be changed. It is not an issue. It is only an issue with men who have agendas other than trying to solve domestic violence. Since ninety-five percent of our cases involve female victims, it makes no sense to give the five percent equal weight. If you say something is gender neutral, you imply fifty-fifty. It's just recently that it has been acknowledged that women have the right to have power in a relationship with men, that men don't have the right to control women. It has been only recently that that consciousness has been on the table, and I'm not interested in finding ways to take it off. Using gender-neutral language would devalue the fight against domestic violence in the overwhelming majority of cases.[28]

This attitude is widespread. It stands to reason that a man seeking help would feel he is not wanted, and cannot be a victim, if the language does not acknowledge his existence. The same reaction would exist for the female offender: "I don't have a problem; it's his problem." This common reaction of male batterers is an attitude that is supported for female offenders by the system.

Would Hess's percentages of male victims in his system change if the language was changed? Probably not, or at least not very much. Much more would have to be done, but the power of language must be acknowledged. Does *gender-neutral* or *gender-inclusive* always imply the current existence of equality? No. The reason for gender-neutral language is to afford an *opportunity* for equality of treatment. Equality does not exist, in fact, without opportunity. It may not ever be possible to achieve equality, and it may not exist in a pure form, but without equality of access, any hope to achieve it is doomed to failure.

Without a sign out front that says, in effect, "You are welcome here, too; we don't discriminate even though you are a minority, and we will enforce a nondiscrimination policy," a minority is unlikely to even seek access; only the very brave will buck the prevailing attitudes. Without such a policy, it is not possible to know how big that minority is or even if it is, in fact, a minority.

For example, what man is going to call the "Women's Crisis Line"? It would be relatively easy to change the name to the "Family Crisis Line," for instance, but few such crisis centers have taken this step. Frequently, there is only one such center for domestic violence help in a given area.

George Gilliand ran for two years what was apparently the only domestic violence shelter exclusively for men in the world, located in St. Paul, Minnesota, in the late 1980s. It eventually closed due to lack of funds. As we have noted, there are now a small number of gender-inclusive shelters serving both female and male victims.

It is instructive to take a look at what Gilliand faced in terms of supporting gender-inclusive language:

> I contacted the county board of commissioners, and in three hours time, I got all of the anti-male literature out of the domestic abuse office. This included a letter from the county attorney that spoke only of helping "you arrest him, restrain him from your home, and keep him away from your children, etc." Within about two weeks after that, I was contacted by the special courts administrator, who had rewritten that letter to gender-neutral language, and he called me down there to approve it. The board later adopted a policy that there would be no literature in the domestic abuse office other than that officially approved. Needless to say, I made instant enemies down there.[29]

He was also able to get the language changed on protective orders. The language in the forms said, "The respondent in this order is the natural/legal father of the below named minor children." He got the language changed from *father* to *natural/legal parent*.

Gilliand started an organization called the Domestic Rights Coalition in 1988. He began to travel around Minnesota, making speeches, creating networks, and talking to court administrators. He says whenever he was in a new area, he would talk to the court administrator about the language in protective orders and get the wording changed. He was successful most of the time, and the language was voluntarily changed, except in his home county. In the 1993 state legislative session, a committee was set up to examine state forms; battered women advocates were invited to attend, but Gilliand was excluded. The language in protective orders was changed, however, and his home county was forced to go along.

We'll have more on the efforts to support gender-inclusive language in domestic violence efforts in the final chapter, but suffice it to say, while there has been substantial improvement, much more work needs to be done.

THE MOVEMENT FOR ABUSED MEN

Who, then, is speaking up for abused men? Warren Farrell, journalist Ellis Cose, and David Thomas in England have written thoughtful and well-documented books that have chapters on the subject. Of particular note for the general reading public is Tom James's *The 12 Things You Aren't Supposed to Know about Domestic Violence*. There are also hundreds of men's groups around the United States and in many other countries.

Nearly all of these groups, however, were organized to deal with issues relating to visitation rights for children, custody rights for men, and in support of joint custody. They may have members who have been abused, and they may express concerns about abused men, but that is not their primary focus. In the 1980s and 1990s the Minnesota group was the only organization with domestic violence against men being a prime concern. Unfortunately, Gilliand's past, including accusations from his children that he was abusive (which he denies), hampers this effort. The first impression I got in my interview with him was how angry he sounded. As he talked, his anger escalated. Author David Thomas noted a similar reaction to Gilliand in his book. I was not greatly surprised, though, at his vehemence. I have talked with many men's groups' leaders around the country, and they don't sound much different. They come to the issues from personal experience with the domestic relations legal system, and this experience has left them bitter.

For the men who have devoted much time and energy to their cause, and who have been in the movement for any length of time, there is another reason for this bitterness that has little to do with the success, or lack of success, of their organization. They are angry at the system, but they are also angry at other men—primarily, the men who call and complain and want assistance but do nothing to help.

The history of the men's movement is fraught with disunity. The contrast with the successes of the women's movement is dramatic. There are many reasons, which are topics for discussion in a different kind of book, and not all can be laid at the feet of the men's groups. The Children's Rights Council in Washington, DC, which takes a very firm gender-neutral approach and has many distinguished women associated with it, has had notable successes in putting on national conferences and increasing public and congressional awareness about visitation access and other issues.

When this book was first published, this section was titled "No" movement for abused men, it is now changed to "The" movement.

Stop Abuse For Everyone, the Domestic Violence Hotline for Men and Women, the National Coalition of Free Men (particularly the Los Angeles Chapter), the San Diego Men's Center, AMEN of Ireland, and the National Family Violence Legislative Resource Center (full-disclosure: the author is on the board of directors) are among the most prominent organizations now promoting the issue. The successes and failures of these groups are discussed in Chapter 5.

MOVING ON

As we have discussed, reaction from women's shelters to the first (and only) TV movie on the subject of men being abused was mostly positive after some initial negative response. At the root of the negative reaction by some feminists to discussing or acknowledging the subject of battered men is a fear that funding for battered women's programs and shelters might be harmed.

I do not believe that loss of funding is a necessary outcome, and Patricia Overberg, the former Executive Director of the Valley Oasis Shelter in Lancaster, California, for one, agrees. She says other shelters can follow her example and provide services for battered men and female perpetrators as well as for women victims and male perpetrators. She says the greatest need is for groups and counseling that do not require in-house shelter. She understands the reluctance to possibly take away funding from a women's shelter by providing a men's shelter and the problems in providing separate facilities; however, a gender-neutral helping approach by crisis lines, counselors, shelter workers, and domestic violence programs would only enhance the effort against all types of domestic violence and not curtail funding.

In our final chapter, we will examine in greater detail possible new or revised approaches to domestic violence in light of a better understanding of its true nature.

Chapter 5

Exploring New Approaches to Reducing Domestic Violence

Much progress has been made in recent years in dealing with domestic violence. Indeed, we have seen that the rate of violence in the home against women has shown a decline, which consistently shows up in the various general population surveys. Feminist organizations, the women's movement, battered women's shelters, and social scientists all deserve a great deal of credit for the decline. It appears that the rate of female violence against men has remained about the same. There is still much to be done to prevent domestic violence against both men and women.

This chapter will look at some fairly new methods in an attempt to address domestic violence. We will also examine some models for prevention. Further consideration will be given to reworking existing programs to deal with the true nature of the majority of domestic violence.

LEGAL IMPROVEMENTS

Mandatory Arrest

A majority of states have mandatory or preferred arrest policies; that is, the victim, who is often afraid to do so, is not required to press charges in order for the offender to be arrested. The responding officer is obligated to make an arrest when there is an apparent physical injury caused by a family member or household member. The fear of imminent serious bodily injury, or circumstances in which the offender purposely forces a person to engage in involuntary sexual relations, can also prompt an arrest.

The law can be clear that police have the authority to determine who the victim is. The officer can determine who the assailant or potential assailant is by considering the seriousness of the threat or threats, the history of domestic violence between the couple, the potential for future assaults, the comparative extent of the parties' injuries, and the possibility that an act was committed in self-defense.

We do not want a policy that arrests both parties when one party is the primary abuse victim, even though both may have been injured. We do want a policy that separates mutually violent couples, which may mean in some circumstances both are arrested. We do need a policy that arrests the prime perpetrator of abuse. This leaves significant discretion in the hands of the officer on the scene, but it is one way to stop further abuse immediately.

Even in areas where this law is on the books, however, some police have not been educated on how to apply it. A number of domestic violence workers around the United States say that, particularly in smaller communities, this law is not enforced. A great deal of education is still necessary, even in large urban areas, to enforce the law on behalf of female victims and even more so for male victims.

Although further research is needed, men who were the subject of a domestic violence complaint were somewhat less likely to reoffend if they were arrested, but chronically aggressive batterers did not seem to be deterred by arrest.[1] Research indicates that a majority of suspects discontinued their aggressive behaviors even without an arrest. This suggests that policies requiring arrest for all suspects may unnecessarily dilute community resources by mandating arrest for all suspects, thus failing to provide specialized and targeted intervention strategies for the worst offenders and those victims most at risk.[2]

Gender-biased application of mandatory arrest law raises serious civil rights issues. Men are arrested, and mandated to batterer intervention programs (BIP), in alarmingly greater numbers compared to women based on known prevalence rates in the population. But it also sends dangerous signals to both men and women in mutually violent relationships. Women may feel absolved of any accountability for aggressive or violent behavior, escaping necessary interventions. Men may become alienated and hostile to a system they believe is stacked against them. Paradoxically, mandatory arrests may disempower victims by taking the decision making out of their hands. The same criticism has been made of no-drop prosecution policies, in which domestic assault cases are prosecuted even if the victim does not want to press charges. Linda Mills, a professor of law and social work at New York University, has written an excellent book on this issue (*Insult to Injury: Rethinking Our Responses to Intimate Abuse*, Princeton University Press, 2006).[3]

Women are more likely not to report a new incidence of violence if, in the original case, the defendant was prosecuted in spite of the victim's wishes, if they believe the justice system failed to enact a "more therapeutic" approach toward the offender, and that as a victim they had no rights or input in the criminal justice system.[4]

Appropriately, our society currently views domestic violence as a crime, not a private matter. However, if in the past battering was often treated as a family squabble, current law frequently treats every family squabble as battering. Instead of a sweeping, one-size-fits-all approach, there should be more differentiation between serious and potentially dangerous cases. More studies are needed on the enforcement and the consequences of mandatory or presumptive arrest policies. Anti–dual-arrest clauses, which often serve as vehicles for gender bias, should be repealed and left to the discretion of the police officers to decide whether there is one primary aggressor, as in stranger assaults, or whether both parties are at fault. Unless the victim is in danger or has suffered serious injury, or children are involved, the victim's wishes not to prosecute should be respected.

The general public may have more realistic view of mandatory or preferred arrest policies than the legislatures that imposed them. During the later part of the Clinton presidency, I conducted a nonscientific person-on-the-street poll, asking these questions of about 40 adult males and females:

1. Have you heard that Hillary Clinton slapped and likely threw a lamp at Bill Clinton after he had to admit the affair with Monica?

The majority of people had not heard of this, but all said in effect, that they were not surprised, and believed it had occurred. Many people laughed and some, mostly women said, "Well, he deserved it."

2. Had it been Hillary having the sexual incidents with a male intern would your reaction be the same if Bill did what she did, that is slap her and throw a lamp? In other words, would she have deserved it?

All of the people questioned stopped laughing, took a more serious tone, said she would not *deserve* it, but said it would be understandable if he reacted this way.

3. I explained that most states have mandatory or preferred arrest laws, and that if anyone was injured in even a minor way, such as Bill having a red visible mark from a hard slap, or a hard object that could cause injury being thrown, that the policy mandates an arrest. The question then became, "Should Hillary Clinton have been arrested?"

All of the people questioned said that she should not have been arrested. All of those questioned said, in effect, that it was likely a one-time thing, understandable under the circumstances, that these kinds of things sometimes happen in a marriage, and the police getting involved would just make things worse.

Initial Response Assessment Team

There is considerable debate over the effectiveness of mandatory arrest laws, the lack of or type of training law enforcement receives in determining primary aggressors, whether dual arrest is warranted or should be used as a tool, and whether the wishes of a victim who does not seek an arrest of a perpetrator should be honored. It may be an unrealistic expectation that law enforcement officers have the time or the training to make effective assessments when initially responding to a domestic dispute. Also, law enforcement officers in many localities do not have access to a database on prior child abuse reports from the domicile.

One way to overcome these obstacles is to have a member of a local Initial Response Assessment Team also respond to the scene. Team members should not be associated with or part of a victim advocacy group or organization. Those associated with local batterer intervention programs could be part of this team if they have adequate training in gender-neutral assessment training and testing, which should be a requirement of BIP personnel in any case. Community professionals with adequate assessment training, and psychologists and certified counselors could also be a part of this team. The cost of such a team should be relatively minimal for most areas, provided that the costs are shared across multiagency lines, that is, sheriff, city police, state police, county/city/state government, district attorney office, judicial district, and so on. Team members should also have access to child abuse reporting agency databases, as well as other databases more commonly available to on-scene law enforcement, such as whether a restraining order has been issued, prior arrest records, and whether there have been prior complaints. Team members can be on-call via pager or other device for rotating assignment for 24-hour coverage. In many areas, a relatively small team can be on-call to respond as needed, be paid less for on-call duties and compensated at a higher rate when actually responding. Liability insurance, waivers, and other needs would be necessary for such a team to be assembled, but these conditions can be met at minimal cost. Team members would receive training by law enforcement in how to proceed without interfering in officer duties, making the assessment process a joint effort with the officer(s) on scene.

Physical danger to the assessment team member should be relatively minimal for two reasons: (1) the team member always allows the officer(s) to secure the scene, and (2) the team member begins the assessment process only when the officer determines it is safe and appropriate for an assessment. Given the research indicating 50 percent of domestic disputes involve mutual non–self-defense combat, and that the majority of cases involve relatively minor physical attacks and victim resistance to appropriate arrest and ultimate prosecution, there is a clear need for more effective and appropriate on-scene assessments and recommendations for the on-scene officer.

Such recommendations may range from arrest to no arrest, involving or not involving child protective services, and dual or single party arrest when warranted. With more fully trained assessment personnel on-scene, alternatives to arrest and prosecution can be contemplated. For example, the officer could issue a citation in a relatively minor family conflict scenario that would mandate that the couple attend and complete a testing assessment of the couple at a later date. With the current availability of family conflict and aggression testing tools and consensual dual polygraph testing, citations for mandatory assessment can result in recommendations to district attorneys and courts with much greater reliability regarding whether prosecution should move forward, upon what basis a restraining order should or should not be issued, and whether child protective services should be involved. In cases where no further official action is warranted, couples would have much improved access to counseling and information regarding preventing similar conflicts in the future. Accurate identification of victims and perpetrators would be more likely and victims would have improved access to information about available resources. Under the further *assessment citation method,* victims would be more likely to assist in prosecution. Each state and locality would have to examine the legal basis for citation mandating assessments. However, in many areas legislation may not be needed, as mandatory assessment could be an added component of existing disturbing the peace statutes.

Whereas an educated and vigorous arrest policy is the most important first step in dealing with domestic violence, our jails and prisons are overcrowded, often resulting in offenders being released prematurely. Although a stay in jail may help to cool things down temporarily, it does not provide long-lasting help for the victim or the perpetrator. Restraining/protective orders usually form the next line of defense for domestic abuse victims.

Restraining/Protective Orders

Restraining orders seem to be of value in protecting people from nonviolent harassment. However, the issuance and enforcement has troubling implications for civil liberties, and greater steps need to be taken to ensure that restraining orders are not used merely as a legal tactic to gain an advantage in divorce/child custody cases.

One solution would be an expedited evidentiary hearing soon after a restraining order is issued. Furthermore, domestic violence victims must be educated about the fact that a restraining order is unlikely to stop a truly dangerous batterer. In extreme cases, criminologist Lawrence Sherman has suggested the equivalent of the "witness protection program"—state-subsidized relocation and resettlement under a new name—for victims who fear for their lives once the abuser is released from jail. Another possibility for consideration is civil detention for particular abusers after they have served a jail or prison sentence, if a review determines that they pose a danger to their victims, akin to the current practice in some jurisdictions of civil detention for dangerous sex offenders. However, such a remedy should be used very cautiously because of obvious potential civil rights problems.

Those civil rights problems are not minor. There has been much discussion and press over what rights terrorism suspects should have. The fact is, that with at least one to two million restraining/protective orders issued against U.S. citizens each year (we don't really know for sure how many), the civil rights issues of these citizens have not been at the forefront of concern.

Several law review articles have pointed out that a proceeding with criminal consequences (up to a year in jail in most jurisdictions for violation of an order) should not be disguised as a civil proceeding. Furthermore, the right to a trial by jury is denied, as is the right to have an attorney if one cannot afford one. The right to call witnesses in one's own defense is frequently denied as is the right to cross-examine witnesses, although a recent Supreme Court decision (Crawford v. Washington (02-9410) 541 U.S. 36 (2004) 147 Wash. 2d 424, 54 P.3d 656, reversed and remanded). has supplied more rights in the area of cross-examination, the right to an attorney if one cannot afford it, or a jury trial is still denied. Notice is a problem as well, even though personal service (rather than just mail) is the norm in most areas. Should the respondent decide to contest the order in a hearing (the only way it can be vacated), they are usually given just two weeks to hire an attorney if they can afford one. Indeed, one might say that the actual effect of such orders is more draconian than many criminal convictions. After all, not only does it carry the potential penalty of jail time, it also frequently means the loss of all possessions, the home, and the loss of contact with one's own children.[5] Comments in the notes by Harvard Law Professor Jeannie Suk in this section are particularly chilling in their implications. This is not only due to civil liberty and legal rights concerns, but she concludes that restraining orders constitute a state-imposed restructuring of intimate relationships.

Courts have little difficulty in issuing protective orders in cases in which there is forensic evidence, police reports, medical records, witnesses, obvious injuries, and other evidence. When there is no such evidence and only the two parties' veracity to determine, courts must err on the side of safety, but should be mindful of the very real possibility that an order may simply be a tactic to gain custody of children and/or possession of a domicile.

We do not know how often this type of abuse of the system and the party named in the order actually occurs. Besides the interviews related to this kind of thing in Chapter 2, I was struck by two cases that came to my attention. In one, a police officer was chosen to be on a panel I participated in on the *Sally Jesse Raphael* television show. He lost his job as a result of a restraining order taken out by his wife, since the order prevented him from carrying a firearm. After the program, I spoke with him and his attorney, and a reporter for *People* magazine (which never did do the story—the reporter later told me it was too "politically incorrect" so it was never done), also interviewed the pair. Although we only interviewed one side, the police officer and his attorney denied the allegation of the "threat" of violence, and it was notable that while the other abused men on the show suffered physical violence, he was the only participant so traumatized by the events that he cried on air. I also interviewed the adult daughter of a woman who was sharing a nice suburban house with her mother. Further inquiry found that neither she nor her mother could really afford the house based on their current income. The house mortgage, however, was free. The daughter explained that her mother was frequently physically abusive to her boyfriend who owned the house. After many incidents (in which he never called police), he finally did strike back at her. She did call police, he was arrested, a restraining order removed him from the house, and she got possession, but he still pays the mortgage. It had been a year since the arrest, the mother contends that she should be compensated for her financial support and half the equity while they lived together, so she lives rent free while the court process drags on.

Mandatory Assessment

In cases where child abuse is not alleged, cases where allegations of abuse are disputed and the court has some doubt as to whether abuse has actually occurred, where the accuser may be the actual perpetrator or it is a case of mutual abuse, the court can follow a policy of ordering temporary mutual shared physical custody of minor children. The couple is then mandated to an assessment. If both parties fail to attend and comply with the assessment, the order is vacated. If only the complainant complies, the order stands. It is not our purpose here to go into great detail about the nature of such an assessment. See *Gender-Inclusive Treatment of Intimate Partner Abuse: A Comprehensive Approach* by J. Hamel (Springer, 2005) for details on practical repeatable assessment tools, and tools used by the Los Angeles Gay & Lesbian STOP Partner Abuse Program for examples.[6] With the advent of such tools, trained assessors in conjunction with consensual dual polygraph testing, the court would have an unbiased, knowledge-based report in which to order a continuance of a restraining/protective order, or to issue a mutual restraining/protective order, and to decide whether one or both parties would retain temporary custody of minor children, or whether only one party should have temporary custody pending the outcome of further litigation.

In less populated areas, the cost of the proposed program could be shared by multiple court jurisdictions, and the assessment team could secure grants by establishing a nonprofit corporation. Although it is desirable that licensed psychologists or other licensed mental health practitioners conduct assessments, licensed individuals could be used in a supervisory role once the program is up and running and highly trained, lower-cost personnel, preferably individuals with additional experience in the field of criminology, could conduct the majority of the assessments.

A few court jurisdictions have begun to move toward granting mostly mutual restraining orders upon first application. There has to be some justification presented at the "emergency" hearing that only one partner needs to be kept away. The mutual order says that *both* parties must stay away from each other, and if either one violates it, that person will be arrested. When children are involved, unless there is an allegation of threat, kidnap, or abuse against a child, temporary custody is made jointly and both parents are given equal time with the child(ren). The exchange of the child(ren) is then ordered to be made in a public place, under supervision, or in the presence of a witness.

Mutual restraint may well be the better method, since it seems to provide the same level of protection as a single-person restraining order yet has less potential for being abused in a custody battle. When the full restraining order hearing is held, if the case can be made that only one of the partners needs to be restrained, then a single-party restraining order can be granted and temporary custody assigned as the judge sees fit.

Some have commented that we need to do away with the whole system of restraining orders due to the great number of problems with the current system: the civil rights issues, the great number of false allegations, the race to the courthouse to see who can get an order first and therefore be the one to remove the other party from the home and get possession of property and custody of children, the fact that they generally fail to prevent a truly violent person from acting, and a host of other problems. I predict that there will be an increase in court challenges to their issuance. Indeed, as of this writing, some have already been started. These criminal cases disguised as civil cases should provide the same protections to the innocent-until-proven-guilty basis of our justice system; the right to a trial by jury if requested, the right to an attorney if one can not afford one, and other common protections offered to the accused in criminal proceedings. The fact remains however, that judges are loath to not issue one upon request. All it takes is a few press reports about one case where was not granted to someone seeking it where they later suffer serious injury or death, and their career is over. My purpose here is to attempt to offer some practical and cost-effective alternatives that can be implemented within the current operating system.

Short jail stays and restraining orders form the primary means of dealing with domestic violence by the law in most areas. The next step is used with far less frequency.

Criminal Charges

Criminal prosecution can be brought by district attorney offices. The problem lies with the scarce resources that many DAs have. It is not pleasant facing a choice between putting time and personnel into prosecuting an armed robber versus a domestic violence criminal, but it is a choice that often must be made. The choice that is most often made is to put the most resources into prosecuting the armed robber or other types of crime (except murder) between nonintimates.

Separating the two people involved in a domestic violence situation is usually seen as the most effective solution to an immediate problem. Putting someone in jail to protect one certain other person is a different type of crime prevention from using the jail to protect a number of potential victims. Thus, jail as a means to deal with violence among intimates takes another step back in the hierarchy of prosecution, even though it can be effective.

These issues reinforce a certain lack of desire by district attorney offices to prosecute owing to their frequent encounters with the primary problem facing them: a lack of cooperation by the victim. The domestic violence victim's frequent failure to prosecute has been documented (see Chapter 1) and is related to the "makeup" period within the dynamics of the syndrome. The victims often return to their abusers. It is no wonder that prosecutors become disenchanted with this type of case. Certainly, prosecutors can proceed without the victim's full cooperation, but it makes for a very difficult case to prove in court. Victim advocates and caring, compassionate prosecutors can be very effective in steering the victim to resources and ultimately preparing and persuading the victim to help them make a criminal case, but this is time-consuming, and the results are more uncertain than other types of criminal cases.

Lack of Legal Representation

If one is a victim of a domestic relations crime, legal help is often needed. Although most courts have clerks that can help a victim fill out a restraining order, the process can be confusing and intimidating. Certainly if a hearing is held on the order and the perpetrator has an attorney and the victim cannot afford one, the victim is at a disadvantage. If there is a divorce or custody case involved as well, legal representation is even more crucial.

The lack of low-cost or free-to-the-indigent legal services is a problem not unique to domestic violence crime. Legal Aid services do exist in many localities, but victims face long delays and overworked staff. As with restraining orders, it is often a case of who gets to the courthouse first. Legal Aid rules prohibit providing representation to both sides in a suit; if the perpetrator applies for representation first, the victim is shut out. Given the unique position of Legal Aid offices, the policy of only representing one side when both sides in a civil domestic law matter are indigent should be reexamined.

In a very few communities, there are sliding-scale nonprofit legal agencies that provide clients with a range of domestic relations law services. These legal practices receive funding from foundations as well as from private donations to make up costs not covered by the sliding-scale fees. The key to providing such services is nonprofit status and an involved board and executive director committed to providing the service and to securing the funding. The need for comprehensive lower-cost legal service for all domestic relations cases is evident in every community. The Bar Association has volunteer lawyer services for the indigent, but domestic relations law is one of the most underrepresented areas in most Bar volunteer efforts.

Community and state domestic relations task forces should concentrate efforts beyond general public awareness campaigns. Making presentations to schools of law and legal associations about the need for, and importance of, assistance to domestic violence victims should be a priority. There is no reason, for instance, why law students could not help those with low incomes with restraining orders and other types of relatively simple legal forms. In many law schools, this is already being done; the students act under the supervision of a licensed attorney and gain practical experience. State laws that inhibit or prohibit paralegals from providing low-cost assistance with legal forms need to be changed.

Judicial Training

In looking at the legal system's approach to domestic violence, a key player cannot be ignored. The ultimate outcome of many cases depends on the attitude and approach of the judge.

It is essential that domestic relations court no longer be treated as a training ground for the least experienced judges. Judges who primarily serve on this court should receive higher pay. Courts need to elevate the prestige of the positions and should insist on continuing education and training in the dynamics of domestic violence and other areas of concern such as child custody and child abuse/neglect. Such training for judges and prosecutors does exist; the problem is that it is not often required or even supported.[7]

Judges must understand that domestic relations/juvenile court is not the least important area in the system, but the *most* important, because an effective judge, implementing and assisting in providing prevention programs, can greatly reduce the overall criminal caseload. If we want to see fewer criminals in our courts, these are the only courts where prevention of the next generation of criminal behavior has a real chance. Court should be the last resort, and society routinely demands that judges solve too many problems. Certainly, the prime emphasis should be on other prevention methods outside of court. If a judge is forced to make a ruling, there is the opportunity, with proper training, to make a real difference for children and the family life of adults before more obvious criminal behavior takes place. Judges in this court must walk a fine line between excessive interference in private matters and judicial activism for society's benefit.

There is an approach that seeks to use criminal prosecution and the use of jails only for what might be termed *hardened* domestic violence perpetrators.

Deferred Sentencing or Batterer Intervention Programs

The deferred sentencing program takes a "carrot and stick" approach to domestic violence. The Duluth, Minnesota, Domestic Violence Project is a national model.

In deferred sentencing, offenders choose to plead guilty to the domestic violence charge (usually a misdemeanor) and to have their sentence put on hold for 6 to 12 months. During this period, the offender is required to participate in counseling and education (depending on the state law, from 24 to 52 weeks). Offenders must report to the probation department. If the offender violates the terms of the program or has another offense, he faces sentencing by the judge and probable jail time. The program is usually limited to those who have not had a prior person-to-person misdemeanor conviction within the last 10 years. Offenders must also be free of any felony convictions, or more than four nonperson misdemeanor convictions, and not have participated in the program before.

At least in theory, this policy is commendable. Researchers, advocates, and professionals who work with abuse victims typically note that the majority of women do not want the relationship to end; rather, they want the abuse to stop. Thus, effective treatment for batterers, preferably coupled with counseling for the victims, would seem like a salutary approach. Yet, the efficacy of these programs has been repeatedly called into question. Some of the findings on the subject are reviewed by Katherine van Wormer, professor of social work at the University of Northern Iowa, and clinical social worker Susan G. Bednar in a 2002 article in *Families in Society: The Journal of Contemporary Human Services*. Van Wormer and Bednar report that a 1987 evaluation found significant reductions in abuse in the first three months of the abuser's participation in the program, and some reductions over a one-year period. A later study, which reviewed the records of 100 former program participants over a five-year period, found a 40 percent recidivism rate. It is worth noting that at least one study cited above reported that 60 to 70 percent of domestic violence offenders did not reoffend *regardless* of criminal justice intervention.

Van Wormer and Bednar also cite a 1991 survey of 76 shelters for battered women on the effects of batterers' programs. Only 12 percent of the respondents reported a decrease in emotional abuse toward women following the men's participation in batterers' programs, while 46 percent saw no impact in this area, and 42 percent reported an *increase* in such behavior.[8]

Batterer treatment programs are rooted in feminist ideology, having close ties with battered women's advocacy groups. Typically, they embrace a model that regards battering as a pattern of coercive control and male domination of women. In such programs, other factors that contribute to violence, that is, psychological, mental, and emotional disorders; drug and alcohol abuse; or violent family dynamics involving both partners, are at best considered of minor importance, or worse, ignored. The focus on *power and control* and male privilege may be the right approach for some abusive men. However, the reality of domestic violence is far more varied and complex. Indeed, in recent years, some who have worked within Duluth-style programs for years, and even those who participated in the design of the model, have candidly admitted the limitations of this approach.

Ellen Pence, one of the creators of the Duluth program, wrote in 1999:

> By determining that the need or desire for power was the motivating force behind battering, we created a conceptual framework that, in fact, did not fit the lived experience of many of the men and women we were working with. The DAIP staff... remained undaunted by the difference in our theory and the actual experiences of those we were working with.... It was the cases themselves that created the chink in each of our theoretical suits of armor. Speaking for myself, I found that many of the men I interviewed did not seem to articulate a desire for power over their partner. Although I relentlessly took every opportunity to point out to men in the groups that they were so motivated and merely in denial, the fact that few men ever articulated such a desire went unnoticed by me and many of my coworkers. Eventually, we realized that we were finding what we had already predetermined to find.... [W]e had to start explaining women's violence toward their partners, lesbian violence, and the violence of men who did not like what they were doing.[9]

The majority of states today establish guidelines for the certification of programs into which the courts may direct domestic violence offenders. In at least 20 states and many smaller jurisdictions, the certification requirements explicitly and specifically include compliance with the feminist model. A 1998 review of 31 sets of standards currently in use in the United States found that "patriarchy is often cited as causing and/or maintaining men's violence against women, or more specifically with the Duluth model."[10] Often, the guidelines also require that programs be monitored and evaluated by battered women's advocates. Methods considered ideologically suspect by the advocates, such as joint counseling for couples in violent relationships or counseling involving other family members, are rejected outright while other approaches such as substance abuse treatment are deemphasized.

For instance, the Massachusetts guidelines state:

> While the following methods may, from time to time, be incorporated into an intervention model that focuses on power and control in relationships, they are inadequate and inappropriate for batterer intervention if they stand alone as the focus of intervention:

>   A. Psychodynamic individual or group therapy, which centers causality of the violence in the past;
>   B. Communication enhancement or anger management techniques, which lay primary causality on anger;
>   C. Systems theory approaches, which treat the violence as a mutually circular process, blaming the victim;
>   D. Addiction counseling models, which identify the violence as an addiction and the victim and children as enabling or co-dependent in the violent drama;
>   E. Family therapy or counseling which places the responsibility for adult behavior on the children;
>   F. Gradual containment and de-escalation of violence;
>   G. Theories or techniques, which identify poor impulse control as the primary cause of the violence;
>   H. Methods, which identify psychopathology on either parties' part as a primary cause of violence;
>   I. Fair fighting techniques, getting in touch with emotions or alternatives to violence.

The guidelines also reject outright the option of couples counseling as a component of batterers' intervention and state that joint counseling should not be permitted until there has been no violence for a minimum of nine months.[11]

In Oregon, state guidelines adopted by the office of Attorney General declare that these intervention methods are "Inappropriate": "Offering, supporting, recommending or using couples, marriage or family counseling, Identifying any of the following as a primary cause...poor impulse control, anger, past experience, unconscious motivations, substance use or abuse, low self-esteem, or mental health problems of either participant or victim."[12]

I've conducted a few nonscientific polls of average people who do not have any particular interest in this issue. When I briefly explain the BIP program and then tell them what is forbidden to be included, their mouths always drop open in astonishment. Let's see: substance abuse, anger, mental illness is not to be considered; couples counseling is prohibited; and licensed counselors are not required. Is the Oregon Attorney General (and other states adopting similar guidelines) just nuts, stupid, doesn't care, or simply uninformed? It would be difficult for the Oregon Attorney General to claim ignorance as he was given a detailed and scientifically based critique of the proposed guidelines that was totally ignored. It would be easy to claim that the attorney generals and legislatures of the states adopting these kinds of guidelines are simply nuts or stupid. Unfortunately, the real answer is more mundane. They put their fingers in the air, saw which way the political winds blew, and recognized that the various state's domestic violence coalitions held the political power of groups concerned with the issue and went along with their concepts. Science lost to ideology.

Ellen Pence of the Duluth Domestic Abuse Intervention Project concedes that in their zeal to counter negative stereotypes of women, many battered women's advocates have fallen into the trap of a "women are saints" mentality: "In many ways, we turned a blind eye to many women's use of violence, their drug use and alcoholism, and their often harsh and violent treatment of their children."[13] Abused lesbians have been the most obvious victims of the battered women's movement's reluctance to confront female violence, which has begun to change only in the past few years. Among heterosexual women, women who are abusive toward spouses or children, or those involved in mutually violent relationships, are unlikely to benefit from interventions that encourage them to see themselves solely as victims.

Given the rise in female arrests, many areas have begun to put into place such programs for female perpetrators as well as male perpetrators. It gets a little confusing, however, given the predominate (Duluth) model; how does male patriarchy fit in? Well, that gets explained to the arrested women as their violence being only a reaction to such male tactics. In some areas, the guidelines state that a male and female counselor must co-jointly present the classes, but for female perpetrators, only women presenters are allowed.

Most states adopting such BIP guidelines do not require that the presenters be licensed mental health practitioners, only that they go through a fairly lengthy training in the predominate model. Thus, the underlying and central problems of many of the mandated do not get addressed. For example, tests for mental illness and substance abuse are not routinely conducted. The charming serial killer Ted Bundy, for example, would sail through such a program undetected.

At a major domestic violence conference, a presenter told the story of the reply received over the telephone for a grant from the National Institute of Justice to study traditional batterer intervention programs as to whether they are effective in reducing repeat offenses. The applicant was told, "No, we already know they don't work." In plain terms, that says it all.

A major review and overhaul of state guidelines for batterer treatment programs is in order, and should contain these essential features:

1. Court-certified abusers' programs should rely on a variety of approaches, including anger management, substance abuse and mental health treatments, couples counseling, and individual counseling that avoids the confrontational, ideological approach of the strict feminist model. Advocacy groups should not have a central role in determining and enforcing the standards for batterers' programs. Instead, states should draw on a diverse community of scholars, mental health professionals, social workers, family counselors, and criminologists.

2. From the beginning of the intake process, batterer intervention programs must have a risk assessment protocol that has as its goal a determination of the level of risk for serious reassault and lethality. Additionally, significant attention needs to be paid to the role of alcohol and other substances in violent offences. The risk assessment is then used, in conjunction with a couple's/family assessment, in order to place individuals and couples/families within a range of treatment and intervention options, or for referral to a Threat Management Team. This function can be assumed by a centralized referring agency, multidisciplinary team, or through single program structure.

3. A couples/family assessment would identify couple/family dynamics that contribute to abuse and violence with the goal of recommending interventions and treatment with attention to couple or family desires.

4. A multidimensional and multitracked treatment system that includes, but is not limited to, same-sex group treatment for men and women, individual psychotherapy, medication evaluations and treatment, group and single couple conjoint counseling, family therapy, inpatient and outpatient substance abuse treatment, and foreign-language cultural specific

interventions that can be mixed or matched with individual, couple, and family needs.

5. Ongoing short-term and long-term follow-up is necessary to identify the continuing intervention needs of couples and families, for outcome and evaluation studies to be conducted on the efficacy of different interventions, and in order to develop a pool of mentoring professionals for those in treatment. Ongoing monitoring should be given priority to those couples or families that have the highest risk of serious violence.

A comprehensive model program, including many assessment tools for professionals, is available in John Hamel's book *Gender-Inclusive Treatment of Intimate Partner Abuse* (Springer, 2005).

In the first edition of this book, the deferred sentencing or batterer intervention program method was discussed and generally supported. The research into such programs had mostly not been conducted, however, and no states had adopted guidelines. Such programs, as least as far as the predominate model is concerned, may simply represent, at best, another case of good intentions gone astray.

These main weapons in the law's battle against domestic violence (arrest, restraining orders, threatened or real criminal charges, mandatory counseling/treatment) can be especially effective if there is communication among the police, district attorney's office, social service providers, and courts.

COORDINATION OF LEGAL AND SOCIAL EFFORTS

Multidisciplinary Task Force

Even within the predominantly women-only services for abuse victims, there is a lack of coordinated effort. In many areas of the United States, efforts are hampered by a lack of awareness of what others are doing, not only in the shelter network but also by police agencies, district attorney offices, social service agencies, probation departments, and the courts. There has been considerable progress made in this area in the last 10 years. It's likely that most areas of the country now have county-level domestic violence coordination councils, which are less cumbersome than statewide councils.

These councils' job is to see that representatives from all agencies are aware of meetings and encouraged to attend, to coordinate funding requests, to implement cross training, to publish a newsletter to all agencies coming in contact with domestic violence, and to promote a public awareness campaign.

Liaisons from the county or metropolitan area task force can help assist communication among all departments; for example, when a restraining order violation appears before a judge, the DA assigned may have very little history on the case because the file is not available or is not complete.

Data Collection

Although individual district attorney offices or police and sheriff departments may collect statistics on domestic violence, it is often the case that these data stay in that office. In other words, a city police department responds to domestic violence calls, but the sheriff's department may also respond to calls within the same metropolitan area. The district attorney's office prosecutes a certain number of cases. All three agencies are dealing with domestic violence, but the numbers are not shared and are often not compiled and collected for a statewide picture of domestic violence. Even if they are collected, different definitions of what constitutes a response call, a complaint, or a report cause confusion due to lack of standardization.

A survey of 44 states found 39 reporting incomplete information, and 33 said there was poor participation from law enforcement agencies.[14]

Some states have moved to correct these problems. The first step is legislation that requires law enforcement agencies to report statistics on domestic disturbances and to prepare quarterly and annual reports to the state. The state agency is then put in charge of collecting these reports and publishing the results that are obtained.

The biggest problem is that without standardization of record keeping among the various law enforcement agencies, even states that collect the statistics and then go the next step to enforce reporting still don't have an accurate picture. This failure has more meaning than simply the desire for a more accurate representation of domestic violence totals because victims are also affected. If an assaulter is brought before a judge on a restraining order violation, the assigned DA may not be aware of more than the one complaint. In reality, police records might show a history of police calls to the residence or to prior residences elsewhere. It is not that this information is unavailable from the police; it is just not available in a timely fashion, given the caseload of the prosecutor's office. Sometimes it is a matter of definition; perhaps the prosecutor looks for domestic violence "complaints" involving the person, but in some jurisdictions a "complaint" means only formal charges, while everything else is a "report."

The domestic violence task force at both local and state levels can help solve local communication problems and improve standardization of reporting methods by assuring that representatives from a wide variety of agencies are working together on common issues. By having more accurate statewide indications of official responses to domestic violence, we can better understand the true cost of those responses, and we can then improve the coordination of resources. If each state standardized data collection and reporting, a more complete and accurate national picture of domestic violence would emerge.

Much progress has been made in these areas in recent years, with the inter-agency sharing of computer records, and record keeping software, but more needs to be done. It is a problem of people and lack of agency cooperation and contact rather than technology.

Family Court

Domestic relations law has one of the highest dropout rates for lawyers and judges. In most courts, the newest and least experienced member gets divorce court. It is not a sought-after area. It is simple human nature and a matter of legal training. In other legal arenas, guilt or innocence is involved; in this arena, there are winners and losers, but no guilt or innocence is determined under no-fault divorce laws. The proceedings are emotionally draining; most murder trials seem simple by comparison. Few involved seem satisfied by the result. In the main, judges are trained to deal with a system set up on an adversarial basis, while judges in domestic relations law are attempting to do the opposite with the people before them and seek to have them quit being adversaries, par-ticularly when there are children involved. Because domestic violence cases fall under the general category of domestic relations, the same judges are usually involved in divorce, custody, and paternity cases.

I have yet to meet a domestic relations attorney or judge (and I have dis-cussed this with many attorneys and judges) who does not agree with this statement: *Domestic relations cases should be taken out of the adversarial court system.* Lawyers are not trained to deal with the psychological and social problems of families. We should not be asking them to do a job they are not trained to do. We should be assisting people to make these decisions for themselves.

There is a model program that began in Sedgwick County, Kansas (Wichita area), where judges no longer hear custody or visitation cases. Instead, the fol-lowing procedures are followed.

Children of Divorce Class

All divorcing couples (including the unmarried who file paternity or affil-iation petitions) who have minor children are required to attend a class on divorce and its effects on children. If there is a restraining order due to abuse, there is an opportunity to take the class at a time when the former partner is not present. The class is funded primarily by participant fees. In some areas, similar classes are paid for by a portion of court filing fees or a combination of participant fees and court money. Reduced fees from the indigent are accepted.

Administration and other small costs are funded by grants and donations to the nonprofit agency holding the classes in a contract with the county.

It is well known that domestic violence often reoccurs when there are children involved, even after a separation. If parents, through a simple and effective course, can be assisted to understand the grave damage that results to their children from physical violence or even verbal arguments, then surely we have made some difference. The focus of the class is on how to avoid involving children in marital conflict and to support a continuation of a dual parenting role. In the more than 40 U.S. jurisdictions where such classes are mandatory, components usually include some instruction on conflict management as well as preparation for mediation and that has a direct bearing on reducing the potential for further or future domestic violence. The Kansas model class is working. There has been a decrease in the number of conflicted domestic relations cases of all types, according to the county's presiding judge.

The chief objection to the idea of the class seems to be that "good" parents who do not have a conflict in their divorce over their children should not be required to attend. Indeed, surveys of those who attend such classes show that most resent being forced to attend. The same surveys show that after the class an overwhelming majority agree it was very valuable and that they probably would not have attended had it not been mandatory. It should also be noted that while many former parenting partners separate amicably initially, trouble often arises later when one or both find new partners.

Mandatory Mediation

As in Sedgwick County, some areas follow the parenting class by mandatory mediation if there continues to be a conflict involving custody or visitation. In most areas of the country where mandatory mediation exists separately or in conjunction with the classes, if a restraining order has been issued, mediation is not mandatory. The rationale behind this is that in a battering situation the abuser is so dominating, intimidating, and controlling that the victim may give away too much to the detriment of self and children. The second point against mandatory custody or visitation mediation for domestic violence cases is the issue of being unable to ensure the safety of the victim. These do not appear to be persuasive arguments when weighed against the benefits of mediation.

Consider these factors. A mediated conference takes place in an environment different from where the abuse occurred. A neutral party is present whose precise job description and training are aimed toward one goal: allowing no one to get the "upper hand." Competently trained mediators are extremely cautious and aware of couple dynamics that may signal dominant and submissive partnership roles. They are trained to seek out true feelings, ask questions, and speak up and act as an advocate for a partner who appears to be dominated. Most mediators have sessions with each party privately, before the individuals are brought together for a joint session. The mediator acts like an interpreter for each side's position. In short, if there is a single profession that is prepared by formal training to counter the typical actions and attitudes of a domineering and controlling spouse, it is a psychologist or a family mediator. Psychologists are too expensive to provide to all separating parents, but we can supply mediators.

Mediators have the added benefit of being results driven. The idea is to come up with a settlement that can be written into law. The outcome is geared toward assisting in reaching an agreement that is acceptable to both sides, yet recognizes that not all areas under contention may be agreed upon. What is not resolved is left to the judge to decide if the two people cannot decide or if their attorneys cannot reach agreement for them. Trained mediators try; they don't pressure. No good system has a quota for mediators in terms of settlement outcomes. If no agreement can be reached, this outcome, too, is accepted.

The safety issue does not hold up, either. There is no absolute safety. If the perpetrator of domestic violence is intent on harming the spouse, the abuse will likely happen. It is less likely to happen at a courthouse or near the courthouse/police station complex, where publicly funded mediation services are usually provided. Mandatory mediation in custody or visitation disputes should be a part of every court system.

There have apparently been no empirical clinical studies of the effects of mandatory mediation in cases where an abusive relationship exists, but we can validly assume that it makes sense to do everything possible to reduce future conflict between separating couples. By reducing the conflict in one area, such as custody and visitation, we will reduce the chances of domestic violence post-separation.

There is no general taxpayer expense involved in mediation. Funding for mediators usually comes from filing fees or sliding-scale fees paid directly by the parents or a combination. Court districts do not even have to hire mediators directly; a coordination person is often sufficient. A rotating list of qualified and scheduled family mediators can come from the professional community. The rotating list is essential. As has been noted, most areas do have county-level mediators, but the quality of the services, according to many, leaves much to be desired. The burnout rate is high. This is understandable. Imagine if it was your job to listen to family personal squabbles day after day. The government pay and benefits are decent enough, but it's understandable if the burnout rate is high. Setting family mediator standards is easy: Meet the qualifications for membership in the American Academy of Family Mediators.

These standards are high and require specialized training in addition to an appropriate educational background.

Court-Imposed Counseling Group

In Sedgwick County, if there is still no agreement between the couple on custody or visitation even after the class and mediation (which eliminates about 90 percent of the court caseload), some couples go to group counseling. The judges assigned to individual cases determine which of the cases are best suited to group counseling and which cases bypass the group process and go to the next step. The groups are usually a mix of men and women. A counselor runs the group and may concentrate further on conflict management skill building, reminders from the class, and other helpful techniques and information. If there is still no settlement, the counselor makes a recommendation to the court.

Custody-Visitation Evaluation

This step is not unique to the Sedgwick County process, as many areas order these types of evaluations by counselors. It is when these evaluations are usually ordered, however, that is the key to the Sedgwick County success. The couple may or may not be involved with the group session before or after this evaluation. Whether an evaluation is conducted depends on the judge's decision based on the record so far. With the knowledge that the couple has at least gone through the class and mediation, and possibly the group session, judges tend to have a more comprehensive record to go by and more certainty that such an evaluation (which can be expensive for the couple) is needed. In many areas, such evaluations are a standard request to the court at the first sign of a conflict, as each side's lawyer attempts to protect the client's interests. Whatever the outcome of that kind of adversarial-based evaluation, it is a certainty that the only winners will be lawyers and the various paid evaluators.

Arbitration

An arbitrator provides a function very similar to that of the mediator, with one important difference: A decision is made. An arbitrator meets with the litigants (perhaps individually first), goes over the main issues still unsettled, explains the law (arbitrators are often attorneys or specifically trained mediators), and tries to help the individuals reach an out-of-court settlement. If there is still no agreement, the arbitrator consults with the judge about points of law and makes a recommendation to the judge. The judge then imposes a ruling on the disputants. The judge is not legally bound to accept the arbitrator's recommendation.

The Sedgwick County system of domestic relations court is the oldest and most comprehensive in the United States to fashion a plan that seeks to remove domestic relations cases as much as possible from the adversarial system.

The good news is that it has been adopted elsewhere—but only in pieces. The mandatory children of divorce class concept has been adopted in some form in most parts of the U.S. local court system. Mandatory mediation for couples in conflict over custody and visitation is even more uniformly applied.

The comprehensive approach involving all elements of the effort, including group counseling, arbitration, and a less-adversarial system of custody/visitation evaluations, is still not very common at all.

Benefits of This System

The Sedgwick County approach makes a great deal more sense than approaches in other jurisdictions. The system has not received much research attention, but it is obvious that it has the potential to provide a number of benefits to society:

- Less stress on children. Children may well be less likely to be involved in abusive relationships themselves when they are adults.
- A vastly reduced caseload for courts, enabling them to spend more resources on criminal matters.
- Less taxpayer expense.
- Parents who are more satisfied with the outcome and thereby less likely to engage in conflict after the separation.

Although most parts of the Sedgwick County system have been in operation since 1980, and at least the parenting class exists in some jurisdictions in nearly 40 states with a few states having it available in every county, and many more areas have stand-alone mandatory mediation, there is a significant gap in these approaches.

SEX ABUSE REVIEW PANEL

Two of the individual cases presented in Chapter 2 were abused men who had allegations of child sexual abuse made against them. Canadian researcher Gregorash found two allegations of abusing children among the abused men she studied. Both men described in Chapter 2 were eventually found innocent. Gregorash did not report the outcome of the charges in her study. The allegations in the two cases presented here appear to be a continuation of the abuse they suffered. It is obvious that in a parental separation case the chances of false allegations being made are greater than in another type of case. Indeed, at least one investigation of court records by psychologists found that in divorce cases about 40 percent of such allegations were false.

The review panel concept has yet to be tested on any widespread basis. More explicitly, it could be called "The Peer Review Panel for Allegations of Child Sexual Abuse in Domestic Relations Cases." Attorney Ron Johnston of Portland, Oregon, has drafted voluntary court papers for this process, but it has not been put to widespread use in that area, and I do not know of many other areas of the country that have used it. This panel would not get involved in criminal cases, nor would it intervene in cases where state child protective services have made firm determinations. It would come into play only in cases where there is not enough evidence to prosecute on criminal charges and where there is not enough evidence to greatly involve state child protective services. The court must consider such allegations seriously when making decisions about visitation and custody, and many DA offices will wait until the domestic relations court's disposition of the case before deciding whether to proceed with criminal charges. In disputed cases, child protective services are often also inclined to wait and take no action, other than perhaps imposing supervised visitation, until after the domestic relations case is adjudicated.

Other problems emerge, however. For one, there is the tremendous expense involved, as both parents, on the recommendation of their attorneys, hire their own clinical psychologists. Second, the child(ren) may be abused by the process itself. In one case, for example, a child was examined and/or interviewed by 12 different psychologists. The case lasted nearly three years. Third, the process sets up clinical psychologists as "hired guns." Lawyers know how to play the game and choose the psychologist that the courts seem to like the best. It may not be the psychologist with the best clinical skills but the one who can do the best job in a courtroom setting. The way out of this problem is for courts to refuse to accept any more hired guns. Instead, this process is followed (simplified here):

Standards. These are set for membership in a professional review panel. The panel will include pediatric physicians, child clinical psychologists, clinical social workers, family nurses, and other experts in the field of child sexual abuse. A larger community liaison group is also formed and holds regular meetings.

Standard order. The court approves an order, which can be implemented on an appropriate case-by-case basis, in which both parties are mandated to cooperate with the panel, turn over all records, and abide by the panel's recommendations.

Record evaluation. The panel appoints a case manager or case managers to evaluate the records and recommend if further evaluations are needed.

Panel discussion. The panel collectively reviews the case and agrees with or changes the case manager's recommendations.

Progress report. The case manager(s) follows the outcome of any further evaluations, reports back to the panel, and recommends further steps, if needed.

Panel decision. If a determination is called for, the panel makes a majority recommendation to the court.

Judge's decision. The judge makes a ruling regarding custody and visitation but is not bound under law by the panel's recommendations.

The cost of the panel's work is paid for in the same manner by which expert testimony is now paid for—by agreement between attorneys or by court ruling; however, because the panel is acting as a collective unit, and sharing expenses, costs should decrease. It certainly represents a much less expensive procedure than the current system of competing experts. In addition, there is the opportunity for lower-income and indigent access to highly competent experts under this system, whereas under the current system, such access is limited or simply not available. The review panel has a greater opportunity than individual private practitioners to get under the umbrella of an existing nonprofit agency (or of forming its own) in order to garner grants and donations to serve the indigent and lower-income and to help with administrative expenses.

The review panel concept would seem to be an appropriate vehicle to test for usefulness in these very difficult cases, particularly when the parents have been involved in domestic violence. There are other beneficial services that should also become more widely available.

SUPPORT GROUPS

Every community should provide support groups for separated parents and for children who have experienced parental separation. Equally important, every community should provide support groups for all victims of domestic violence. Sharing common experiences truly works wonders toward helping individuals rebuild shattered lives.

SUPERVISED VISITATION SERVICES

Every community should provide three types of services:

Site-specific. A secure facility service is needed where visitation is monitored when there has been a sufficiently believable allegation involving abusive behavior directed at the child by the visiting parent, or at the other parent in the presence of the child, or in which there is a serious threat of parental abduction. In some cases, even supervised visitation is not allowed by the court.

Off-site monitoring. Off-site monitoring provides a means by which a supervising monitor may go with the child and visiting parent to public places conducive to parental and child interaction. This service provides a more natural setting, as well as a certain level of child and parental protection.

Visitation exchange. Visitation exchange provides a neutral party to the visitation exchange of children in cases involving allegations of abusive behavior directed at one of the parents. The Children's Rights Council now has set up a number of visitation exchange centers. The monitor's presence is usually enough to inhibit such conduct. A monitor also acts as a credible witness to the court. The parents normally understand this, so abusive behavior is less likely. This service is of particular benefit to victims of domestic violence, because controlling behavior, verbal and/or physical abuse, has an opportunity for renewed occurrence during visitation pickup and delivery.

Visitation monitors need not be expensive. Their job is simply to provide a safety presence. They should not provide reports based on parent-child interaction; that is the role of counselors and psychologists. Visitation monitor reports are limited to a simple statement of what happened and whether any specifically inappropriate or prohibited behavior took place.

Trained volunteers can certainly be used for visitation exchange monitoring and can also help with off-site and site-specific monitoring. The services can be provided by existing social service and nonprofit agencies. A modest expenditure of public funds or fee collections can be used to supplement the budgets of such agencies.

The steps outlined here to provide resources for separating parents are needed in many types of cases. Being mindful of the child's needs as well as the parent's is the cornerstone for successful implementation of such programs. We can now turn our attention to other reforms that should prove beneficial for abused persons whether or not there are children involved.

SHELTERS

First, there does not appear to be a widespread need for shelter services for battered men, except in large metropolitan areas, because until there is an increased awareness that violence by men's mates is as wrong as battering women, men will not seek to gain access to such shelters.

Update: When that sentence was written 10 years ago, it was a valid recommendation. It is no longer true. The rise in arrest rates for women alone, and the increased awareness of the issue, now means that there should be a shelter to accommodate abused men and their children in every area that has one for women.

It is, yes, a civil-rights issue. Assuming that at the lowest possible end, 25 percent of the victims of domestic violence are heterosexual and gay men. Should we deny them services available to others merely because of their gender and sexual orientation?

The answer still seems to be, yes we should. Consider, for example, the United Way, the largest charity-dispensing agency in the United States. It has denied funding the Boy Scouts of America because the Scouts will not hire gay scoutmasters. The United Way charter prevents it from funding organizations that practice sexual discrimination. The United Way is one of the biggest givers of funds to the YWCA. The YWCA runs the largest, and by most accounts, some of the best anti-domestic violence service centers in the United States. It, of course, discriminates against men. Is there a domestic violence program of equal stature at the YMCA? No, there is not. Has the YWCA across the country demonstrated many efforts to also offer services to men? You already know the answer.

I continue to fear a struggle over funding at a time in which some battered women's shelters are turning away many applicants for shelter because of a lack of space. The last thing we need to do is increase the battle between men's rights and women's rights groups by escalating a social service battle over scarce funds. Primary efforts should be concentrated on funding different and mainly preventative approaches to domestic violence, which have the potential of reducing the need for more shelters for women or men.

Third, a primary purpose of women's shelters is to provide a safe place that prevents homelessness for the indigent. Shelters often provide up to a 30-day stay and help locate further transitional housing. The fact that men rather than women make up the overwhelming majority of the homeless is an argument for making transitional housing available for the abused male. Most homeless programs recognized this reality, with the result that there are more homeless beds available for men than for women.

For the abused male forced to leave home who does not have children, there is a statistical economic advantage over his female counterpart—the potential for a 22 percent greater income. The U.S. Census Bureau, on the other hand, finds that for unmarried, single women without children ages 18–34, there is near wage parity, with women earning just two cents less per dollar than men on average, but for all working women of all ages, women who work full-time earn 78 percent of what men earn.[15] Still, on average, there is a greater opportunity for a man to secure transitional housing and temporary shelter due to his gender than there is for a single woman.

When children are involved, the picture changes dramatically for both men and women. At shelters, one of the greatest needs is for adequate and appropriate facilities for children. It is also more difficult to locate transitional housing when children are present. Employment assistance is more difficult, and affordable day care is also difficult to find. When men leave an abusive home, they may be less likely to have children with them than are women. This is changing, as more men become primary caretakers of children. Our priorities in providing shelter space for men with children should reflect societal changes and individual circumstances. Until awareness of male abuse by both victims and shelter providers improves, little can be done to ascertain what the need is for space for men that also accommodates children.

The human picture tells us that there are a number of abused men with and without children who do not fit the average. Are we to ignore their pain and suffering simply because they are a minority? Shelters do more than simply offer a temporary place to stay; they offer hope, support, and counseling specifically targeted to the victims of domestic violence.

The numbers may not support providing as many shelters for men as for women, but the numbers are sufficient to demonstrate a need in most areas for such shelter. When women's shelters first began, officialdom said there was not a need; the need became apparent only after the shelters opened. It is impossible to know for certain the level of need until after such shelters become more established for men.

Some shelters do accept male victims but only because they also serve as shelters for the homeless. The level of outreach to male victims of domestic violence at this type of institution is not very high. Of those shelters that specifically serve both men and women, the overall numbers of men being sheltered are much less than the number of women helped in this manner. Valley Oasis provides a series of cottages for both men and women. Thus, they have spaces available that can be separated by gender.

Even shelters that are in one house or building, with a little creative thinking and reconfiguration, can accommodate a few men as some have found out, with separate entrances, a room that can be locked off from the rest of the house as the need arises, and so on. (Note: It was one of the most thrilling moments I had in doing the second edition of the book to change the tense of that sentence to reflect that the number of shelters serving men and women in one location has indeed increased from none to nearly a dozen taking the exact approach described here.) As new shelters are opened or remodeled, of course, a simple consideration of the practical needs of abused males and their children can be incorporated in design decisions without interfering with or threatening female residents.

It is certainly true that any shelter that can only accommodate women can at least provide hotel vouchers for men. Most shelters already use this method when they do not have the space for more female residents.

CRISIS LINES

It is very clear that crisis lines that address men's particular needs and concerns should be established. The producer for *Men Don't Tell* noted that there was not, at the time, a toll-free number anywhere for men or their friends and relatives to call to get information. Now, DAHMW exists, and SAFE operates a non–toll-free number for information about services around the country. AMEN in Ireland now operates a similar service in the UK.

However, all of these organizations suffer from underfunding, and at least in the United States, it is unlikely that you will find their numbers in a medical clinic office card or even publicized on most domestic violence organizations' Web sites. The National Coalition Against Domestic Violence Hotline squarely occupies the position. It has apparently never made the effort to find out who on its referral list actually serves men. Indeed, the organization and hotline has done little to promote any recognition of their plight.

On the other hand, there is no reason that local domestic violence crisis lines cannot handle calls from both male and female domestic violence victims. Jan Dimmitt is the executive director of the Emergency Support Shelter of Kelso, Washington. Like the Valley Oasis Shelter of Lancaster, California, her organization fields calls from both women and men seeking help. While this shelter does not currently provide housing services for men, it does help them when they call. Dimmitt says setting up this effort was difficult:

> My feeling is that we are not touching the tip of the iceberg by our domestic violence programs as we see them today. We talk exclusively of women. The road to enlightenment has been a rocky one. Whenever I speak of male abuse, I am met with disbelief and, even worse, laughter. We are looked upon as being friends of the perpetrators rather than friends of the victims, because all males are supposed to be evil and bad. If I mention [to staff] that we have a woman in here that deserves to be charged, rather than counted as a victim, I then become the bad guy. I notice in talking with other shelter staff throughout the state that attitude prevails in the other shelters, too—men are the perpetrators, women are the victims.
>
> When I have answered the phone myself, which I don't do very often, I have had a number of calls from battered males. In one case I recall, a man had been out drinking and came home to fall asleep on the couch. His wife took an iron skillet and beat him. He was admitted to the emergency room of the hospital and stitched up. He was taken there by the police, but no charges were filed against his wife. My heart goes out to the men who call because there are no services available for them, other than with a psychologist or psychiatrist. I have some doubts about many of them [therapists] as I feel they are back in the dark ages of how they stereotypically view males.

However, some progress has been made in that we are now making contact with all victims of domestic violence and employ a male to make the initial contact with the men. He tries to be an advocacy-based counselor for them, and that was a giant stride. We do help them fill out protection orders, and we do go to court with them as a friend and supporter, just as we do for female victims. If they need immediate shelter we refer them to a local shelter that is for all homeless people, but that lacks the services available for female victims in that there is no support group, and no individual counseling.[16]

Still, in a growing number of areas, there is now a place to call. There is no reason why the expertise, training, and understanding developed at crisis lines for female victims cannot be used to help male victims, even if full shelter services are not available.

All it takes is a change in attitude, and sometimes a slight name change (i.e., Women's Crisis Line to Family Crisis Line or Beth's House to Family House).

There are some hopeful signs. Writing in *The New Yorker,* Luis Menand spoke to the core issue:

> Violence can be talked about in the abstract, but violence, like sex, never occurs in the abstract. It is always a conjunction of singularities. We have fallen into the belief that morality can be ascribed to groups. But groups cannot be moral or immoral: "Women" are not more or less moral than "men."... Morality is an attribute only of persons. Individuals can suffer because of the group they are perceived to belong to, and they can benefit by identifying consciously with a group, but no one is a better person simply by virtue of belonging to a group. Groups are essentially imaginary. Souls are real, and they can be saved, or lost, only one at a time.[17]

The road to enlightenment is indeed a rocky one, but that must not prevent us from trying. If the current shelter and crisis line system for domestic violence persists in denying even simple services to male victims and female perpetrators, there are and will continue to be further lawsuits over discrimination in funding.

VIOLENCE AGAINST WOMEN ACT

Even though there was an indication of congressional intent in the original passage of the Violence Against Women Act (VAWA) that males could be served by funding, during the first five years of the act, there simply was not; in fact, some facilities seeking to serve men were denied funding. That was changed in the third reauthorization with specific language allowing funding for services to abused men. The interpretation of the language change, however, by the Office of Violence Against Women is that funding for male victims will only go to programs that "primarily" help women. Thus to get a share of federal funds under VAWA, one can set up a shelter and/or crisis line exclusively for women, but not one for men.

Perhaps even more important, the General Accounting Office was directed to find out something about the effectiveness of programs, how the money is being spent, and who is being served. The first GAO report basically said that the system of reporting was so bad, it could not answer these questions. The second report was a little better (at least in terms of determining who was being served by the federal money—only 10% men), but there was little in terms of detailing outcome effectiveness and determining how the money was spent. The name of the law needs to be changed, perhaps to something like "The Family Violence Act."

A detailed critique of VAWA compiled by Respecting Accuracy in Domestic Abuse Reporting (RADAR) is included in the Appendix.

At the state level, the prediction 10 years ago about lawsuits, has turned out to be true. The Third District Court of Appeal in Sacramento has ruled California's exclusion of men from domestic violence violates men's constitutional equal protection rights.[18]

The taxpayer lawsuit was initially filed in 2005 by four male victims of domestic violence. In 2007, Sacramento Superior Court Judge Lloyd Connelly dismissed the case, ruling that men are not entitled to equal protection regarding domestic violence because they statistically are not similarly situated with women.

The Court of Appeal *reversed* that decision and held: "The gender classifications in Health and Safety Code section 124250 and Penal Code section 13823.15, that provide state funding of domestic violence programs that offer services only to women and their children, but not to men, violate equal protection." This ruling could (depending on each state's constitution, laws, and regulations) provide a persuasive argument for similar lawsuits in other states.

My hope is that there will not be a need to battle in the legal arena for a protracted period of time in different areas; this would only add to the group-against-group mentality that Menand eloquently wrote about. No matter what the numbers are of men needing these services, we should not discriminate on the basis of gender or minority status. If there is just one abused man or woman perpetrator out there in need, we should help.

CAUSES

Domestic violence cannot be separated from its causes. The causes have more to do with societal and personality issues that are distinctly different from issues of relations between men and women.

TV and Movie Violence

Television and movie violence is one of the areas commonly cited as contributing to domestic violence. Entertainment media violence does contribute to domestic violence in terms of desensitizing some children and adults to the effects of non-make-believe violence, as studies show the greatest effect of TV violence to be one of perception regarding how much violence there actually is in society. Heavy TV viewers tend to overestimate the amount of violence. The extent of a direct cause-and-effect relationship between violence viewing and violent actions remains under investigation. To the extent, however, that parents can limit more impressionable children from viewing movie and TV violence, every effort should be made to do so. Enough studies exist (and enough advertising is bought to prove it) showing that TV exerts a powerful influence, both good and evil. There should be no stinting of efforts to influence the entertainment arts that domestic violence is a subject worthy of attention, but the present gender-biased double standard should be eliminated. Domestic violence against men should not be treated as humorous or deserved in entertainment scripts. The same approach and sensitivity to the issue should prevail for both sexes.

Isolation

Isolation of the family from kin, neighbors, and community is seen as another contributing factor. Economic pressures have resulted in a mobile society. It takes time to build a sense of community and neighborhood. It takes a certain enabling stability to access community resources that help a couple or family under stress. Domestic life is under assault by rapid change. The old neighborhood is not there anymore. Relatives are scattered across the country, and strangers live next door. Given the fact that domestic violence by its very nature is a mostly hidden crime, and its occurrence is likely to contribute to a couple or family becoming more insular, the increased isolation of each of us from one another facilitates the continuation of this form of violence.

One opportunity to mitigate the isolation takes the form of a concern that is supported by the media (and is even sensationalized) and can form a common bond in neighborhoods where everyone is a virtual stranger: crime. We can use this concern over "outside crime" to form neighborhood bonds and help overcome isolation. A program as simple and effective as Neighborhood Watch has been shown to overcome years of isolation among neighbors. Indeed, it is not unusual for neighbors to meet formally for the first time at these small anti-crime meetings. A community policing program with citizen involvement, which is now in place in a number of localities, has also been highly effective in this regard.

The principal aim of such programs is also met: They do reduce overall crime rates. Preventative in nature, they cost less and provide continuing long-term benefits that may also subtly act to reduce domestic violence by simply helping neighbors become more concerned about each other.

Sexism

Sexism exists and persists. Stereotypes haunt and wound all of us. History is replete with stories of women and men who did not "fit in" to traditional roles. There is a benefit to unconventionality—it often produces our leaders. This is further proof that it is possible to change. The time is ripe for a new marketplace of ideas that features more thoughtful advocates for a changed role between men and women. You can hear them yourself in Jack Kammer's *Good Will toward Men,* a book that consists entirely of interviews with women. Featured are Karen DeCrow, former president of the National Organization of Women (NOW); Barbara Dority, cofounder and cochair of the Northwest Feminist Anti-Censorship Taskforce (NW-FACT); journalist Ruth Shalit; and a number of other influential feminists, including Sue Steinmetz, whose work is featured in this book. Author Warren Farrell in *The Myth of Male Power* has also written about the "second stage" of relations between men and women and their advocates where fairness is the guide. Columnist and author Cathy Young, author Christina Hoff Sommers, Ifeminist.net, run by Wendy McElroy, columnist and author Kathleen Parker, lecturer and victim advocate Stanley Green, Jill Murray Ph.D., author and Vice-Provost at New York University, and others too numerous to mention have taken up the call for fairness and equity. There also appears to be a slow but steady movement within the Gay, Lesbian, Bi, and Transgendered community to recognize that discrimination exists on many levels within the current predominate structure of domestic violence services.

Perhaps more important in the long run, more people in the social scientist, legal, academic, law enforcement, and medical community are taking time to join with others to call for a more scientific approach that includes outcome measurements, best practices, and less ideology. An organization I co-founded, the National Family Violence Legislative Resource Center, is one among several others that seeks to bring together these diverse elements and find common ground in fact-based research and practical application of it for legislation and legal practices. People are finding, somewhat to their surprise, once they find the courage to speak up, that they have more friends than they suspected.

Let me relate one very personal example of this. There are other examples of some fairly well-known social scientists who have experienced similar "conversions." However, I've only met a few of them. I did meet Don Dutton, Ph.D., twice.

The first time was at the domestic violence conference 10 years ago where the really big guy got in my face for handing out a flyer (I had permission!)

about the first edition of this book. The intent of this person (I later found out he is a physician at a large medical teaching college, who was embarrassed enough about his threatening physical action to hide his name tag) was to get me out of the conference. Dutton was a featured speaker.

There's no question that Dutton was then, and is now, one of the preeminent international domestic violence scientists. He has been widely published and his research is a source of reference in the field. After his presentation, I merely came up to him and shook his hand and thanked him for sending me an article of his about gay male victims. He was gracious enough.

However, during his presentation, I noticed that he clicked his PowerPoint slides deliberately past the Straus/Gelles data charts that showed male victims in comparison to female victims. His presentation as a whole only focused on female victims and male perpetrators and never mentioned male victims nor mutual abuse. He seemed to be taking the position voiced by another prominent social scientist, "Well, they only asked me to speak about female victims so that's all I'm going to talk about."

Ten years later we were at another conference, in which I was also presenting. We had dinner later with a group of other people. I did not ask him about the process he went through in the preceding 10 years and why now he was adamantly choosing to recognize and even promote the data about abused men and mutual combat in his presentation. He gave his own story in a very public way. Essentially, he simply could no longer choose to not mention all the evidence available to any group, regardless of any fears of peer pressure or fewer speaking engagements or backlash at his university or other types of consequences. Science won over the politics of fear.

All of these people, and slowly growing number of others, see the opportunity for holding on to a modern definition of feminism that is for equality rather than victimology. It is a movement of inclusion rather than exclusion. It is a healthier movement than it has been, as so many battles have been won against oppression (which is not to say that there isn't much more to be done). It has proven itself as a liberating force for women and men. We have a chance to pause and reassess the focus of these efforts by operating in a less emotional climate. These voices—which have always been there—now have a better chance of being heard. Isn't that the point? Listening first—instead of reacting.

If we can free ourselves of the bonds of what we are "supposed" to be like as men and women—men are independent, forceful, physically tough, good at sports, fearless, emotionally controlled, and nonnurturing, while women are emotional, bad at sports, passive, weaker than men, dependent, and always nurturing—then we can have a movement *and* a home life that sees ourselves first as human beings and only secondarily as two genders. Freeing ourselves of the haunting and hurtful stereotypes of our upbringing is not an easy task. Accepting responsibility for the choices we make is never easy.

We *can* take concrete steps to make acceptance of responsibility more likely and sexism less likely.

EDUCATION

Education is the keystone of reform. All the experts I have interviewed say the same thing: "fund educational programs." They do not mean educational programs solely about domestic violence. They outline a plan for parenting and human relationship education at official, private, social service, and school levels. The ultimate goal is to break the cycle of dysfunctional and violent families.

Although biology plays a role, we have begun to recognize that alcoholism and drug addiction, abused children, teenage parents, poverty, crime, lack of education, suicide, and domestic violence—most of society's ills—are more the result of a poorly constructed family life than of anything else. Strengthening families must be our first priority, or every other kind of effort is ultimately made in vain.

What kinds of educational programs for the family and professionals interacting with families should we undertake? What message should they impart? How can government or quasi-governmental bodies provide what is needed without intruding unduly into private lives, and how do we fund them?

Law Enforcement Education

There are several well-recognized domestic violence training programs available to police. The programs geared toward understanding female abuse victims need to be reviewed for prevention of sexist bias against male victims. The biggest problem—even though it is in their own best interest to deal most effectively with a dangerous situation—is making sure that all law enforcement departments require the courses, and that accurate scientifically based information is being provided.

It is essential that law enforcement officers on the scene have readily available literature and phone numbers for social service and helping agencies related to domestic violence. Coordination among agencies and areas is essential in the provision of these services for all communities.

Teacher Education

Bias against girls in the classroom has been documented by several researchers. The validity of some of these findings has been called into question by author Christina Hoff Sommers. Psychologist Ashton Trice examined 1,200 schoolchildren and found that boys aspire to lower-prestige careers than do girls, and low-income girls tend to have higher career expectations than do low-income boys. Until age 9, suicide rates for girls and boys are equal, but from ages 10 to 14, boys commit suicide at a rate twice as high as girls, and from ages 15 to 19, at a rate four times higher. More women are now graduating from college than are men.[19]

All of these findings indicate that we had best be cautious in attempting to overcome what is perceived to be an unfair advantage of boys over girls in the classroom. It is not easy to resist stereotypes that assume unfairness against only one gender, just as it is not easy to overcome thinking of a boy who is not good at sports, emotionally sensitive, nonaggressive, or more interested in arts than in science as "strange." We do need teacher education that reduces sexist "pigeonholing" for both genders and offers a more balanced view of the gender-oriented classroom research available.

School Classes

Schools cannot solve all of society's problems. In a sense, we already demand too much from schools and have abdicated too much parental responsibility. Nevertheless, the opportunity to reduce interpersonal violence is available to schools, as is the opportunity to educate the next generation of parents more effectively.

We desperately need a class in all schools that goes beyond what is commonly offered. The "Life Sciences" curriculum needs to be a required course for high school, and elements of it should be integrated into all grade levels with changes that are age-appropriate. Such a course should teach the elements briefly outlined here:

- Conflict management skills.
- Interpersonal communication skills.
- Household finance and investment management.
- Job resume, interview, and job-finding skills.
- Work ethic enhancement.
- Ethical choice discussions and activities.
- Anti-violence discussions of media images.
- Effective drug and alcohol abuse education.
- Responsible sexuality.
- For high school students, parenting education with real-life assignments that effectively demonstrate the responsibilities that parents must assume. At a minimum, it must also focus on nonviolent discipline techniques, shared duties between the genders, nutrition and physical health, education encouragement, and ethical parenting choice discussions based on practical life lessons.
- Parental and peer involvement in the program.

Some schools have some elements of such a program already in place. Project Stop, a conflict management program, is in place in more than 30 New York City schools. A program called "Do the Right Thing" has been shown to be quite effective in many schools at reducing physical conflict in school and encouraging good communication skills about personal conflicts. Denver psychologist Carla Garrity and four coauthors have produced a guide for schools called "Bully-Proofing Your School." This program goes far beyond suspending and disciplining bullies when identified. It is a comprehensive program involving staff, parents, and students that enhances caring instead of aggression. West Albany High School in Oregon reduced its dropout rate by a significant percentage when it restructured its class schedule and a staff team was put together to help students with personal, social, and academic problems. Peer mediation, tutoring, and counseling are available. In Silver Springs, Maryland, the Equal Partners program emphasizes self-esteem building, stress reduction, realistic expectations about future goals, and relationship understanding, among other components. Parents are involved in the program. Family and Schools Together (FAST) of Madison, Wisconsin, helps children whom teachers have identified as at-risk for later problems. This program empowers parents to become primary prevention agents for their own children by increasing parental awareness of substance abuse and its impact and by offering a support group for parents. Activities include family communication exercises and winning-as-a-family-unit exercises.

It is not that proven and effective methods are not available or that many schools are not trying to incorporate some of these methods; what is lacking is a comprehensive approach that touches all grade levels and is required within the curriculum.

A significant finding in favor of this type of comprehensive approach was published in 1994 in the *Journal of the American Medical Association*. Researchers evaluated a drug and alcohol abuse prevention program that does much more than simply teach facts about health and criminal dangers; in fact, most of the program deals with other areas. Specifically, these are decision making, self-directed behavior change, coping with anxiety, and social skill building. Booster sessions are conducted so that the entire program lasts over three grade levels for teenagers. The difference between the Life Skills Training Program developed at Cornell University Medical College and other substance abuse programs is that it has been evaluated as effective. School-based programs that focus only on scare tactics and provision of information have not been proven to be effective at prevention of drug/alcohol abuse by teenagers.[20]

The Fast Track program developed at Vanderbilt University has also been shown to be effective at reducing chronic aggressive behavior problems. One critical key to success has been aggressive recruitment of parental involvement.

The lesson from all these programs is clear: To prevent abuse and other social problems that are detrimental to academic and social functioning, use a long-term approach that involves parents, peers, and teachers in a comprehensive program that teaches practical social skills that enhance self-esteem.

Public Education

We have already discussed the mandatory parenting education program for legally separating couples with minor children. Because this course contains conflict management skill teaching, it can do much to reduce domestic violence between these couples as well as help their children and themselves deal more effectively with the trauma of parental separation during and after the fact. Beyond this program, we need to launch a public awareness campaign that is more expansive than solely the focus on battered women. We need to send this message out: People Aren't for Hitting! We need to break the cycle of the most important predictor of domestic violence (besides age), the violent family. We need to do more to publicize the help lines and agencies for child abuse and domestic violence. We need a comprehensive educational program that in short, simple language imparts practical and proven techniques. The media can do much more, although NBC's "The More You Know" public awareness campaign is a wonderful example of the type of program that is needed, but many more such efforts are needed. The public will respond in time by watching, listening, and reading.

Effective, simple, easily understandable, and nonviolent child discipline techniques have been identified by Thomas Phelan's 1–2–3 *Magic,* and others. (This book and available video is highly recommended. I've had parents come to me with tears of thanks in their eyes after implementing the program with their spouse and, as the book cover photo indicates, turning a "monster" child into a happy child.) Shared parenting and responsibility can also be promoted. Conflict management techniques can be easily demonstrated, and interpersonal communication techniques that enhance the self-esteem of adults and children can be demonstrated and taught.

There is no reason that these skills cannot be promoted one at a time. The cumulative effect of this knowledge will be extraordinary.

This skill-based awareness campaign must be supplemented with full-length affordable and available classes. Schools should act to promote and make available adult parenting classes. Governmental and nongovernment agencies can also help to provide and promote education in these areas. Income-based sliding-scale fees should be the norm so that there is not an undue burden on taxpayers or agencies.

Further public awareness of the prevalence of all forms of family violence is needed. Some basic messages must be conveyed: Even one slap is wrong; sibling violence is not acceptable; physical child discipline is not necessary; dominating and controlling your mate is wrong and not necessary; all families and pairings have problems and stresses that can lead to violence; violence in the home is more common than we assume; and mutual violence is much more common than we assume.

THE FAMILY ADVOCACY CENTER

Earlier in this chapter, we spoke of the need for domestic violence coordinating councils and the need for coordination and communication among various official agencies. This is only the first step. The model for a new approach to most forms of family violence and abuse is in place. While it can be put into operation in metropolitan areas most easily, its very existence will greatly help the level of coordination, cooperation, and education in less populated areas. It is founded on the principles that should govern all our actions in regard to home violence, both public and private: Live together. Listen and share instead of reacting and acting in isolation.

Major Emil Daggy of the Marion County Sheriff's Department of Indianapolis, Indiana, is one of the founders of the Family Advocacy Center, which began operation in 1990. At the time, there were no other similar comprehensive operations elsewhere in the United States. City and county law enforcement specialists, physical and sexual abuse specialists from the state child welfare office, and domestic violence and sex abuse prosecutors from the district attorney's office all share the same building. In Indianapolis, about 75 people are employed at the center. In the main, these public positions are not new. They already existed within law enforcement, district attorney, and child welfare departments. What is new is the level of cooperation and coordination. The Family Advocacy Center also employs five people in a private nonprofit agency to help coordinate services among government and private agencies, secure funding, provide education services, and promote public awareness. Standardization of education is a key component. Investigators in both police and child welfare have similar educational backgrounds and training.

Another aspect of the effort is adult services in which police and prosecutors coordinate investigations of domestic violence and elderly abuse—that is, law enforcement, prosecutors, social service agencies, family welfare agencies, and victims' advocates are all communicating with one another. Although victims' advocates, crisis hotlines, and shelter systems are not in the same building, the official agencies share an information system about each case. Daggy has seen a decrease in cases in which the victim fails to cooperate with prosecution. He also sees a more effective system of cooperation and communication among victim advocates from law enforcement, prosecution, and shelters. The nonprofit agency helps outside services coordinate their efforts with officials.

A computerized management information system is in the process of being established. This system means that every case file can be updated by different official agencies. For example, when the police respond to a domestic violence call at a residence, in the past the police would not know that child welfare may have had a report of child abuse at that residence. Child welfare may not have known in investigating a neglect case that domestic violence has also been reported. The new system will allow every agency to enter each report, which will then be shared with other officials. In this manner, a more complete picture of family problems emerges. Agency budgets are more likely to be focused, and duplication of efforts among departments is reduced. In turn, resources to help the family members can be better utilized.

Progress is being made to implement the Indianapolis management information system into a statewide network of standardized data and information sharing regarding all types of family problems.

The key to the center's success is as simple as putting various official agencies concerned with helping combat family problems under one roof. Daggy says this is essential not only for government agencies but also for a cooperative effort with other outside agencies:

> As the center has developed over the years, we have been working very hard to make the center a focus in the community for family violence. Social service providers are involved. We invite them to meetings, get their input, inform them about programs, and process. It wasn't that way in the past. I was involved in a task force commission on youth and families before the center, but they did nothing. They spun their wheels, because they weren't connected with any of the other service providers in the community that did things for kids. So they had no reason to listen or come to the meetings. The center is actively involved in these areas, so it's in the service providers' own self-interest to be involved.

Daggy says there's another benefit of having various agencies under one roof and having a nonprofit agency coordinate improved training:

> The overall training of everybody here is much higher. I've been to a lot of seminars around the country. I've talked to a lot of other people from police departments [and] health care providers; and the level of training here is better than in most communities. This, just because we are co-located and we try to coordinate our efforts. Also because the [nonprofit] Advocacy Center can try to go out and try to get private funding, we have access to more training than we would through normal budgets.[21]

The emphasis of the center is to treat the family as a unit, where one kind of problem is not isolated from another. Daggy says the emphasis is on helping victims and perpetrators: "The domestic violence perpetrators need to understand why they are doing what they are doing, and how to control their tempers, but there are also some dynamics for the victim. They may come from a family where this is the norm, or they have really low self-esteem so they think no one else would like them, so they'd better stick with what they've got."

Daggy points out that while the figures may vary, it is well known that the majority of people in trouble with the law come from abusive families. He says it makes sense to treat the entire family and to look at a variety of issues regardless of the reason for the initial call to officials. He says it is important to bring a variety of resources to that effort in a cohesive fashion:

> There are a lot of people in every community who want to help children, families, battered spouses; they all want to do the same thing, but they're all going in different directions. In most communities there isn't a lack of people who are interested; there is a lack of people going in the same direction. The best achievement of the Advocacy Center is getting people going in the same direction, and treating the family as a total unit.

Unfortunately, the one-stop center for all family problems Indianapolis model is not the program that the majority of federal domestic violence money has actually gone to in the last 10 years. A somewhat similar model adopted by San Diego District Attorney Casey Gwinn got the lion's share of the money for replication elsewhere in the country. It is not that the San Diego program does not have at its core the central services and communication component for domestic violence needs, but it is not as comprehensive as the Indianapolis model in involving more agencies and players in dealing with a wide range of related family problems. I must admit to some bias in evaluating these two models, because Gwinn has expressed doubt in a number of ways on the need of more services or attention for abused men. On the other hand, it is good to see that the efforts to create a more user-friendly and cooperative effort among various agencies using the vehicle of co-location to some degree is being taken seriously and proving to have a range of benefits.

WHAT WE DON'T KNOW

Canadian researcher Lesley Gregorash has interviewed a number of male victims of domestic violence. In the resulting paper, she calls for new research in a number of areas:

> First, it is important to have a clearer understanding of what males constitute as abusiveness, since it appears that vagueness about definition may have led to excessive tolerance of violent behaviors. Cultural approval of violence in

sports and in media requires ongoing research, to determine what impact there may be on men's tolerance of violence against them.

Second, more attention to male needs for attachment in intimate relationships with women is important. This focus should also encompass enhanced understanding of male views on sexuality and its importance to them in relationships. [Note: Gregorash's interview subjects, like many of the men I interviewed, believed that their partners set the sexual agenda, and used access to intimacy as a means of exercising power and control.]

Third, focus on understanding male conceptions of parental roles and the meaning of parenthood is vital. It may be that men want greater involvement in their children's lives, but are limited by traditional notions that mothers should be the primary caretakers.

This society places stereotypical importance on certain resources which men should obtain because they are male (occupational status, income, power through prestige). There needs to be more research about the resources men perceive themselves to be contributing to their intimate relationships, and the reasons they consider these resources important.

Finally, it is important to know clearly what men want from women to feel empowered and nurtured within their intimate relationships.[22]

Beyond these areas, I suggest these specific needs for further research:

1. Nationally representative hospital domestic violence emergency room surveys that include both women and men need to be undertaken, beyond the Justice Department survey that looked at just injury assaults. The surveys should ask questions about the reason for treatment that day; the cause of the injury; whether there had been injury to the other partner; the extent of the injury; and the treatment given, including what further resources the victim was referred to. The surveys should also look at hospital and general care physician response to both male and female victims and then compare these responses.

2. A survey needs to be conducted of family therapists regarding male victimization. We need to discover whether it is true what many male victims and some counselors report: a bias against believing that male victimization exists, not asking questions about male abuse, and seeking change in abusive relationships only in the male rather than treating the family as a system.

3. Although there has been an increase in research, much more needs to be learned about violence in same-sex relationships.

4. Outcome measurements are needed for all types of domestic violence programs and services.

TOWARD A NEW APPROACH

Restoring and strengthening the family should be the focus of our efforts. We will not come to grips with domestic violence against men or women, nor most of the other problems affecting society, without focusing on helping the dysfunctional family in a more coordinated, cooperative, scientific, and preventative way.

We need to free ourselves of the mind-set that sees our own issues as the most important issues, our own agenda as the only agenda, that divides us into competing groups, and that only serves to blind us to the interconnectedness of problems and solutions.

The Introduction mentions my fear that some groups might trumpet the findings presented here, while others might denounce the conclusions. Indeed, as this second edition demonstrates, this is exactly what has occurred. The "ridicule" component, however, has declined. In my first interview with Bill O'Reilly of the Fox News Network, it was, for example, quite apparent that ridicule of the mere existence of men abused by female partners was the main agenda, or at least, great doubt. The second interview was very different as the producers independently came across some research and the interview turned mainly on the issue of just how extensive the problem really is for men, but the ridicule and severe doubt were no longer present. O'Reilly is simply typical in his reaction. The news media only reflect predominate public opinion, so much has changed in the last 10 years. My hope remains that this work will continue to be a launching pad for rational discussion. If it helps to create a greater awareness of the complex issues involved in intimate partner violence and if it helps to support and expand new resources and direct help for abused men and their partners, and improve services to women, as well as gay and lesbian partners, then it will have succeeded. To some extent this has indeed occurred, but much remains to be done.

The research shows us that some form of physical or verbal abuse may be almost as common as love in a significant number of intimate relationships. This finding does not mean that we should stop trying to love or that we should assume the family is a bankrupt concept. If we can move forward to a better understanding of the benevolent and malevolent natures of each gender, we can increase the opportunity for constructive rather than destructive relationships.

Domestic Violence and Injury— The Spread of False Information: Results from a National Survey of Governmental and Large Private Organizations

Philip W. Cook

NOTES ABOUT THIS SURVEY AND HOW IT WAS CONDUCTED

The survey was completed in August 2006. Therefore, it is highly likely that the Internet links to the listed organizations and their statements have been altered since that time. The reader should not rely on the links for a connection but would likely find more value in using a search engine to locate the listed organization to discover what the current statement might be.

How the Survey Was Conducted

One hundred sixteen organizations and prominent individuals were surveyed regarding whether they made a public statement or listed as factual the statement: *Domestic Violence Is the Leading Cause of Injury to Women.*

The statement is false:

The Centers for Disease Control: "National Hospital Ambulatory Medical Care Survey: 1992 Emergency Department Summary" shows that the leading cause of injury, to both women and men, is accidental falls, followed by motor vehicle accidents. According to the CDC, 13.6 percent of injuries to women seen in emergency rooms are from car accidents—a total of nearly 2 million, or almost 10 times the number of injuries from domestic violence. Twice as many women visit emergency rooms due to being injured by an animal (459,000 a year) than by a male partner.

Survey Rationale

To discover the extent and nature of major governmental and large private organizations and highly prominent individuals disseminating false health information to the general public. In particular, regarding a statement that should be apparently false to even an undergraduate in the health care professions. That such a statement was being (and in many cases still is) given as factual by many prominent public health agencies, including the U.S. Department of Health and Human Services, state and local health agencies, as well as the president of the United States, and many other law enforcement, legal, social service, and office holders, should give cause for concern. The discovery that the dissemination of this false health information was widespread and long-lived (e.g., in the case of the U.S. Department of Health and Human Services, it was posted on its Web site and presumably in other publications for eight years) should also be of concern.

This should be of interest to public health administrators and educators, governmental and private agencies, sociologists, and all persons who have an interest in false public health information delivered by public agencies and officials.

Survey Limitations

The survey was limited to discovering whether the listed organization or official made a false statement for public dissemination regarding the extent of physical injury to women as a result of domestic violence. There were several types of variations on the general statement made; in a majority of cases, the false information was qualified to a certain extent by the age range of women said to suffer this injury, although this qualification was also false. The wording of the false statement is noted for each of the listed groups or individuals. Where it was given by those surveyed, the source of the information that they disseminated is listed. In all but three instances given as a source by these organizations or individuals (Stark and Flitcraft 1985, the staff report of the committee on the Judiciary—according to the survey, the two least commonly quoted source authorities—and the National Coalition Against Domestic Violence), the source given never made the statement.

The survey did not, except in a few cases, attempt to examine further news media dissemination of the false data, although a cursory examination of some news media outlets indicates that it may be extensive.

Implications for Future Research

It is hoped that the survey may prompt further inquiries into how widespread the phenomena might be regarding other types of false statements by these organizations and officials. It would also be particularly useful to discover other false statements by these groups regarding domestic violence and compare and contrast such statements with other health-related statements by the same group. Such further inquiry should be able to indicate whether false health information is more likely regarding domestic violence information compared to other public health issues. Certainly an expansion of the survey to include other public agencies regarding this statement and perhaps other false statements regarding domestic violence would prove useful.

THE SURVEY

Alabama Coalition Against Domestic Violence [1]
http://www.acadv.org/facts.html

Alameda Times Star, Alameda/Oakland, CA [1]
http://www.timesstar.com/Stories/0,1413,125~1486~2434345,00.html

Allaboutcounseling.com [4]
http://www.allaboutcounseling.com/domestic_violence.htm

Altria Corporation [2]
http://www.altria.com/media/03_04_03_02_DVBackgrounder.asp

American College of Emergency Physicians, Pennsylvania Chapter [2]
http://www.paacep.org/communications.htm

American College of Surgeons [2]
http://www.facs.org/fellows_info/statements/st-32.html

American Federation of State, County and Municipal Employees [2]
http://www.afscme.org/about/resolute/2002/r35-007.htm

American Institute on Domestic Violence [2]
www.aidv-usa.com

America On Line [1]
http://members.aol.com/butterfly0582/page5.html [2]

Arizona, State of, Department of Public Safety [3]
http://www.azvictims.com/domestic/default.asp

Athealth.com [2]
http://www.athealth.com/Consumer/disorders/DomViolFacts.html

Ayanna Safe Haven, Sacramento, CA [2]
http://maatinus.com/ash/fact_stat_1.htm

Baby Center, The, LLC [2]
http://www.babycenter.com/topic/pregnancy/pregnancysex/1356253

BIOMedcentral.com
http://www.biomedcentral.com/1528-4042/4/179/abstract

Brain Injury Association of America [4]
http://www.biausa.org/word.files.to.pdf/good.pdfs/domestic.violence.pdf

Brush, Colorado, Police Department [3/5]
http://www.brushcolo.com/forum.htm

California, University of, at San Francisco, School of Dentistry, Division of
    Behavioral Sciences [2]
http://www.ucsf.edu/daybreak/1997/11/1124_stu.htm

California State Employees Association [4]
http://www.calcsea.org/csd/committees/women/women_domestic.asp

Callam County Courts, Port Angeles, WA [1]
http://www.clallam.net/Courts/html/court_domesticviolence.htm

Casa Esperanza, St. Paul, MN [4]
http://www.casadeesperanza.org/en/aboutdviolence.htmlDe

Childbirth Solutions, Inc. [2]
http://www.childbirthsolutions.com/articles/issues/violence/index.php

Clark County Sheriff, Clark County, WA [2]
http://www.clark.wa.gov/sheriff/community/domestic.html

Clark County Prosecuting Attorney, Jeffersonville, IN [6]
http://www.clarkprosecutor.org/html/domviol/facts.htm

Clinton, Bill, President [11]
http://www.findarticles.com/p/articles/mi_m2889/is_n40_v34/ai_21275668

Communications Workers Union, UK [3]
http://www.cwu.org/default.asp?Step=4&pid=207

Compass of Carolina, Greenville, SC [4]
http://www.compassofcarolina.org/family_violence_pages/domestic_
    violence_facts.html

Connecticut Department of Public Health [2]
http://www.dph.state.ct.us/OPPE/sha99/intentional_injuries.htm

Cornell University, School of Industrial and Labor Relations [2]
http://www.ilr.cornell.edu/laborAndUnions/UL560.html

DeKalb County Sheriff's Office, Georgia [2]
http://www.dekalbsheriff.org/dvd.htm

Delaware Department of Labor [3]
http://www.delawareworks.com/divisions/dcw/domestic.htm

Domestic Abuse Women's Network, Tukwila, WA [2]
http://www.dawnonline.org/frame10.html?frame10=dv_facts.html

Domestic Violence Center of Howard County, Columbia, MD [2]
http://users.erols.com/cucc/domvioctr.html

Domestic Violence Coordinating Council, Modesto, CA [4]
http://www.co.stanislaus.ca.us/dvcc/content/

Eastside Domestic Violence Council, Seattle, WA [8]
http://www.edvp.org/statistics.htm

Eaton County Prosecuting Attorney, Eaton County, MI [4]
http://www.eatoncounty.org/prosecutor/domesticviolence.htm

Encyclopaedia Britannica, Women in American History [2]
http://search.eb.com/women/articles/domestic_violence.html

Eugene, Oregon, City Police [4]
http://www.ci.eugene.or.us/police/Comm_Policing/crime_prev/domestic.htm

Family Violence Law Center, Oakland, CA [4]
http://www.fvlc.org/gethelp.html

Florida, State of, Department of Law Enforcement [2]
http://www.fdle.state.fl.us/cjst/publications/Rights_and_Remedies/En
   glish.htm

Freudenthal, David, Governor of Wyoming [4]
http://wyoming.gov/governor/press_releases/execorder/2001/domestic
   violence.html

Georgia, State of, Department of Human Resources [11]
http://health.state.ga.us/pdfs/micounsel/violence.96.pdf

Giuliani, Rudolph, Letter from Mayor of New York, 1996 [2]
http://www.nyc.gov/html/rwg/html/96/violence.html

Gotomydoc.com [2]
http://www.gotomydoc.com/education/violence/learn/domestic/

Grohol, John, M.D. [4]
http://psychcentral.com/library/domestic_violence.htm

Hamilton County, District Attorney, Chattanooga, TN [10]
http://da.chattanooga.net/domvio02.html

Harbor Communities Overcoming Violence, Chelsea, MA [13]
http://www.harborcov.org/pages/domestic_violence/index.asp

Haverbrush, Thomas, M.D., Alama, MI [2]
http://www.orthopodsurgeon.com/factoid_farm.html

Health Resources and Services Administration (HHS Division) [7]
http://bphc.hrsa.gov/OMWH/domesticviolence.htm

Idaho Council on Domestic Violence [4]
http://www2.state.id.us/crimevictim/news/news.cfm?category=3&chapter=
30&article=27

Idaho Falls, Idaho, Police Department [4]
http://www.ci.idaho-falls.id.us/main/index2.asp?PageId=492

Indiana University School of Law [4]
http://www.law.indiana.edu/pop/domestic_violence/mythsfacts.shtml

ivillage [2]
http://pages.ivillage.com/debi_1111/id30.html

Journal of Undergraduate Nursing Scholarship, University of Arizona [4]
http://juns.nursing.arizona.edu/articles/Fall%202003/masington.htm

Julien Center, The [4]
http://www.juliancenter.org/more_facts.html

Kentucky University of, Cooperative Extension Service [4]
http://www.ca.uky.edu/fcs/AREAS/Health/newsletter/October_2004pdf.pdf

KERA-TV Dallas, TX [2]
http://www.kera.org/community/breakingthesilence/facts.lasso

Lancaster County, Pennsylvania, Domestic Violence Services [3]
http://www.caplanc.org/factsaboutdomviolence.htm

Lapdonline.org [4]
http://www.lapdonline.org/bldg_safer_comms/gi_domestic_violence/
domestic_myths.htm

Louisiana, State of, Office of Attorney General [2]
http://www.ag.state.la.us/violence/statistics.htm

Maricopa County Department of Public Health, Phoenix, AZ [2]
http://www.maricopa.gov/public_health/domestic.asp

Maricopa Association of Governments, Domestic Violence Council [3]
http://www.mag.maricopa.gov/dv/About_DV/Myths_and_Facts/myths_
and_facts.html

Medem, Inc. [2]
http://www.medem.com/MedLB/article_detaillb.cfm?article_ID=ZZZA
LLZX9FC&sub_cat=2007

Memorial Hospital and Health System, South Bend, IN [1]
http://www.qualityoflife.org/ich/dove/dove1.cfm

Modern Religion, The, Islam [2]
http://www.themodernreligion.com/women/w_violence.htm

Montana Association of Churches Assembly [5]
http://home.earthlink.net/~admassist/violence.htm

Morella, Connie R., M.D. [4]
Congressional Record 10/4/1994

Multnomah County, Oregon [14]
http://www.co.multnomah.or.us/dchs/dv/dvman_whatis.shtml

National Association of School Resource Officers [8]
http://www.nasro.org/members/lessons/domesticviolencestofer.doc

National Library of Medicine, National Center for Biotechnology Information, PubMed [3]
http://www.ncbi.nlm.nih.gov/entrez/query.fcgi?db=pubmed&cmd=Display
&dopt=pubmed_pubmed&from_uid=10540691

National Women's Health Information Center
http://www.4woman.gov/violence/index.htm

Netwellness (University of Cincinnati, Ohio State University, Case Western Reserve University) [2]
http://www.netwellness.org/healthtopics/domesticv/

New Hampshire Coalition Against Domestic and Sexual Violence [1]
http://www.newbeginningsnh.org/html/dv_dv.html

New York State Department of Health [4]
http://www.health.state.ny.us/nysdoh/injury/24_25.htm

Nursing Network on Violence Against Women [2]
http://www.nnvawi.org/conferences_last.htm "A leading cause…"

Oracle Education Foundation [2]
http://library.thinkquest.org/11644/thinkquest_violence.html

Oregon, State of Department of Health and Humans Services, Adult and Family Services
http://www.dhs.state.or.us/abuse/archive/dvnewsletters/dvnews01.pdf

Pataki, George, Governor of New York [2/5]
http://www.state.ny.us/governor/press/oct14_97.html

Praxis International [2]
http://www.praxisinternational.org/downloads/

Price, David (D-North Carolina) [4]
Congressional Record 10/4/94

Puyallup, Washington County of, City Attorney [4]
http://www.ci.puyallup.wa.us/domesticviolence.htm

Quigley House, Clay County, FL [4]
http://www.casnet.com/nfc/quigley/qfacts.html

Safe Passages, Northampton, MA [3]
http://www.safepass.org/two.html

Safe Place, A, Lake County Crisis Center, Waukegan IL [4]
http://www.asafeplaceforhelp.org/domesticviolencefacts.html

San Bernardino County Sheriff, California [1]
http://www.co.san-bernardino.ca.us/sheriff/dvra/dom_viol_facts_main.
    htm

Seattle, City of, Domestic and Sexual Violence Prevention Office [2]
http://www.ci.seattle.wa.us/humanservices/dv/dvinfo.htm

Sedgwick County, Wichita, KS, Office of District Attorney [6]
http://www.sedgwickcounty.org/District_Attorney/dvfactsheet.html

Snowe, Olympia (R-Maine) [3] (according to Surgeon General and AMA)
Congressional Record 10/4/1994

South Carolina, State of, Department of Social Services [3]
http://www.state.sc.us/dss/aps/fv.htm

Spring, The, of Tampa Bay, FL [4]
http://www.thespring.org/main.asp?ID=53

State House Girls Resources, LLC [2]
http://www.shgresources.com/resources/dv/

St. Joseph County, Indiana, Police Department [3]
http://www.in-map.net/counties/STJOSEPH/GOVERNMENT/Stjoesheriff/
    domestic.html

Tauscher, Ellen O., Congresswoman, 10th Dist. CA [2]
http://www.house.gov/tauscher/3-5-99.htm

Teen Challenge International [2]
http://www.teenchallenge.com/index.cfm?domesticviolenceID=1&doc_id=332

Tennessee Association of Alcohol & Drug Abuse Services [2]
http://www.tnclearinghouse.com/factsheets/DVFacts.htm

Trinity University Department of Sociology, San Antonio, TX [4]
http://www.trinity.edu/~mkearl/fam-viol.html

Tulare County District Attorney, Visalia, CA [4]
http://www.da-tulareco.org/domestic_violence.htm

United Nations Commission on Human Rights [9]
UN Department of Public Information DPI/1772/HR Feb. 1996
http://www.un.org/rights/dpi1772e.htm

United Way of Central New Mexico [3]
http://www.uwcnm.org/information/domesticviolence.htm

U.S. Air Force, Air Combat Command [1]
http://www2.acc.af.mil/accnews/oct02/02382.html

U.S. Army, Military District of Washington, DC [1]
http://www.mdw.army.mil/news/breaking_the_domestic_violence_pattern.html

U.S. Department of Health and Human Services, Administration for Children and Families [2]
http://www.acf.dhhs.gov/programs/opa/facts/domsvio.htm

Valley General Hospital, Monroe, WA [4]
http://www.valleygeneral.com

Webmagic.com, Inc.—Abuse.com [1]
http://www2.webmagic.com/abuse.com/index2.html

Westside Health Authority, Chicago, IL [2]
http://www.ebvonline.org/DomesticCM.htm

West Virginia Coalition Against Domestic Violence [12]
http://www.wvcadv.org/health.htm

Wisconsin, State of, Department of Health and Family Services [4]
http://dhfs.wisconsin.gov/womenshealth/WomensHealth/Domestic
Violence.htm

Women's Crisis Center, Brattleboro, VT [1]
http://www.womenscrisiscenter.net/stats.htm

Women's Shelter Program, San Luis Obispo County, CA [4]
http://www.womenssheltterslo.org/info_statistics.htm

Workforce Development Group 1 (claims 1999 UCR)
http://www.workforcedevelopmentgroup.com/news_twenty_three.html

Wyden, Ron, U.S. Senator, Oregon [2]
Congressional Record, Domestic Violence Identification and Referral Act,
Senate, March 14, 1997

Yakima County, Yakima, WA [2]
www.co.yakima.wa.us/Pa/DomVio/DV.pdf

YWCA, Central Alabama [3]
http://www.ywcabham.org/DVRes/safetyplan.asp

Statements by Reference #1–14

Domestic violence is the leading cause of injury to women between ages 15 and 44 in the United States—more than car accidents, muggings, and rapes combined.—According to: Uniform Crime Reports (UCR), Federal Bureau of Investigation, 1991 OR—According to FBI OR—Leading Cause of Injury According to FBI OR—According to U.S. Justice Department. [1]

Domestic Violence is the leading cause of injury to women. [2]

between the ages of 15 to 44. [3]

(and) more common (more often) than automobile accidents, muggings, and rapes combined. [4]

with According to: findings by the former U.S. Surgeon General (sometimes given as Novello or Koop). OR According to Centers for Disease Control OR National Coalition Against Domestic Violence. [5]

Domestic violence is the leading cause of injury to women between the ages of 15 and 44 in the United States; more than car accidents, muggings, and rapes combined. According to: Violence Against Women, "A Majority Staff Report," Committee on the Judiciary, United States Senate, 102nd Congress, October 1992, p. 3. [6]

It is a leading cause of injury to women between the ages of 16 and 44 and a principal reason for women's visits to emergency rooms or doctors' offices. [7]

The Surgeon General stated that Domestic Violence is the leading cause of injury to American women between the ages of 15 and 54. (The Uniform Crime Report, 1996.) [8]

Domestic violence is the leading cause of injury among women of reproductive age in the United States. [9]

Domestic violence is the leading cause of injury to women between the ages of 25 to 44, more common than combined auto accidents, muggings, and rapes (Surgeon General 1992). [10]

A leading cause of injury to American women. [11]

Domestic Violence is the leading cause of serious injury to American women. (Stark and Flitcraft 1985). Referring to E. Stark and A. Flitcraft, "Spouse Abuse," in *Surgeon General's Workshop on Violence and Public Health: Source Book* (Leesburg, VA: GPO, 1985). Also see, *Journal of the American Medical Association* 267, no. 23 (June 17, 1992:3190). [12]

For women between 15 and 44, domestic violence is the leading cause of injury—more common than car accidents, muggings, and *cancer* deaths combined. [13]

Domestic violence is the single greatest cause of injury to women in this country. [14]

Notes

The U.S. Department of Health and Human Services has stated that "Domestic Violence is the leading cause of injury to women." HHS has given no source for this information, and as of June 2005, has removed this statement. HHS has been directly cited by Altria Corporation and many others as the source for this statement. The HHS statement has been used with or without attribution as support for the false statements about injury rates and domestic violence variously attributed to others such as the FBI's Uniform Crime Report, which *has never stated in any year* that DV is a or the leading cause of injury nor that it is more common than car accidents, and muggings, or both combined.

THE TRUTH

The Centers for Disease Control: "National Hospital Ambulatory Medical Care Survey: 1992 Emergency Department Summary" shows that the leading cause of injury, to both women and men, is accidental falls, followed by motor vehicle accidents. According to the CDC, 13.6 percent of injuries to women seen in emergency rooms are from car accidents—a total of nearly 2 million, or almost 10 times the number of injuries from domestic violence. Twice as many women visit emergency rooms due to being injured by an animal (459,000 a year) than by a male partner.

In addition, the most recent U.S. Justice Department Survey (NCJ-156921) of injury-related visits to emergency rooms found that *all* violence is responsible for 3 percent of such visits and domestic violence for 1 percent. In total this means that domestic violence accounts for fewer than 0.3 percent of ER visits. Despite careful charting procedures, it is true that the relationship to the assailant was unknown for one-fifth of the female patients and fully one-third of the male assault violence victims who represented 14 percent and 3 percent, respectively, of all intimate partner assault victims in the national sample (79 hospital) survey. Even if, however, the assumption is made that all of the unknown relationship assault victims were included as domestic violence, it still would not even be close to true that the numbers approach 30 percent of all hospital admissions ("We do know that 20 to 30 percent of the injuries that send women to the emergency room stem from physical abuse by their partners"—former HHS Secretary Donna Shalala, statement to American Medical Association) nor that domestic violence is the single or most significant cause of injury to women or men.

The following study is the one cited by Surgeon General Novello, and then referenced by others. It refers only to one "poor, urban, black community in western Philadelphia, Pennsylvania." Falls exceeded violence as a cause for injury to women of all ages. Violence (but not specifically domestic violence) was the leading cause of injury from ages 15–44. Novello never stated that domestic violence is the leading cause of injury to women in the United States nor among women ages 15–44:

> Although injuries are the number one cause of death for women under age 45 years in the United States, very little is known about nonfatal injuries to women, particularly those from urban, black communities. The Philadelphia Injury Prevention Program is a surveillance system of fatal and nonfatal injuries in a poor, urban, black community in western Philadelphia, Pennsylvania. Nearly 10% of the estimated population of 31,032 women aged 15 years and older suffered an injury resulting in an emergency room visit or death during the 1-year study period from March 1, 1987 through February 29, 1988. The major causes of injury were falls (25.1 per 1,000 women), violence (20.8 per 1,000 women), and motor vehicle incidents (16.8 per 1,000 women). Violence was the leading cause of injury for women aged 15–44 years and the most common cause of injuries among women with two or more injuries during the 1-year period. Injury rates were highest for women aged 25–34 years (157.1 per 1,000 women); nearly 16% of the population in this age group suffered an injury resulting in an emergency room visit or death during the 1-year study period. Rates declined with advancing age for each injury type except for falls, which were most common in young women aged 25–34 years (28.4 per 1,000 women) and in those aged 65 years and older (29.0 per 1,000 women). We conclude that in this population, injuries to young women appear to be a major public health problem. More work is needed to understand the nature of injuries occurring to young women in urban communities.

The full article reference is J. A. Grisso, A. R. Wishner, D. F. Schwarz, B. A. Weene, J. H. Holmes, and R. L. Sutton, *American Journal of Epidemiology* 134, no. 1 (1991): 59–68. The study was conducted by the Clinical Epidemiology Unit, University of Pennsylvania School of Medicine, Philadelphia 19104, http://aje.oupjournals.org/cgi/content/abstract/134/1/59.

Next is a representative example from the survey of a Web page from the American College of Emergency Physicians making the false public health statement. The Web page was examined in August 2003.

Examining this Web page in detail supports the possible conclusion that false, misleading, incomplete, or not useful statements about domestic violence by prominent health organizations are not limited to those related to injury to women. The further false statements by ACEP are so noted at the end of this text.

ACEP Statement: "For help, victims of domestic violence should talk to their physicians or call the National Domestic Violence Hotline at 1–800–799–SAFE."

Fact: The NDVH does not provide help to *all* victims of domestic violence. Its practice is to refer callers to a local agency for actual assistance. The majority of such referrals are limited to helping only women, and therefore do not provide assistance to heterosexual and gay males.

ACEP Statement: "Domestic violence is the single largest cause of injury to women between the ages of 15 and 44 in the United States, more than muggings, car accidents, and rapes combined. Each year between 2 million and 4 million women are battered, and 2,000 of these battered women will die of their injuries."

Fact: As so noted, the first sentence is false. The second sentence is also false, as well as misleading and incomplete.

The only large national survey (although it has been replicated on smaller population samples nearly 200 times) resulting in a figure of between "2 million and 4 million" women affected by domestic violence is the National Family Violence Survey conducted in 1978 and 1988 by the National Family Laboratory Center at the University of New Hampshire and funded by the National Institute of Health. *Battering* by definition means more than a one-time occurrence. This survey only measured instances that occurred "at least once in the last year." It did not measure further frequency of the attacks. Secondly, while it is true that nearly 4 million women a year were affected by domestic violence, this includes what the researchers defined as *minor* violence—a one-time event including only "To throw something at another; to push, grab, shove, or spank." Those in the severe violence category were limited to 2 million women. The statement is misleading as it leaves out important information that the same survey found an equal number of male victims. Failing to mention that males also suffer homicide at the hands of their domestic partners is misleading. More recent large national surveys indicate that the rate of severe intimate partner violence is declining among women from those found in 1988 and no longer equals 2 million women a year. Most notably, the National Violence Against Women Survey (CDC and Justice Dept. funded) found 1.5 million female victims and 885,000 male victims per year in the United States. Murder rates vary year to year, but it is true that the number of female domestic partner homicides has remained near the 2,000 victims a year level. Failing to mention that the male murder rate in these cases averages roughly 25 percent lower is misleading.

ACEP Statement: "Violence against women is an urgent public health problem with devastating consequences for women, children, and families."

Fact: Violence against men is an urgent health problem as well, whether by their intimate partners or certainly in the case of overall criminal violence, which is a larger problem for men. The devastating consequences are also equal for men, children, and families. Indeed, the majority of the perpetrators of child abuse are women:

ACEP Statement: "There is no typical victim. Domestic violence occurs among all ages, races, and socioeconomic classes. It occurs in families of all educational backgrounds."

Fact: The majority of published peer-reviewed research (see http://www. csulb.edu/~mfiebert/assault.htm for an annotated bibliography) has identified a "typical" victim or who makes up the majority of victims: (1) under the age of 35; (2) come from a lower-than-average socioeconomic background; (3) have experienced or witnessed minor to severe domestic violence in their family of origin; (4) they and/or their partner use alcohol; (5) mutual abuse predominates with fully 50 percent of all incidents resulting in mutual abuse, 25 percent of the attacks carried out only by male perpetrators, and 25 percent of the attacks carried out by female perpetrators, with initiation of the attack (who struck first) being equally distributed between male and female partners.

ACEP Statement: "Every emergency department should have written material with the names and telephone numbers of local shelters, advocacy groups and legal assistance to give to patients if they feel it is safe to take it."

Implications for policy: Although this statement is a suggestion to emergency departments, it does carry the weight of their lead organization. It is a fact that few such departments carry any written literature (though it is available in brochure form through SAFE www.safe4all.org) or referral numbers that have any value to male victims.

AGENDA FOR VAWA REFORM

The following agenda is taken from Respecting Accuracy in Domestic Abuse Reporting (RADAR), http://www.mediaradar.org/, and used by permission.

Reducing Partner Violence, Respecting Civil Liberties, and Protecting the Family

Thirteen years after its passage in 1994, the Violence Against Women Act has been found to be *ineffective* in curbing domestic violence, *disrespectful* of fundamental civil liberties, and *harmful* to the institution of the family:

1. A recent review of VAWA-sponsored treatment programs and law enforcement strategies found that most programs were ineffective in curbing abuse, and some of them are actually harmful.[1] For example, a recent

Harvard University study of mandatory arrest policies concluded, "intimate partner homicides *increased* by about 60% in states with mandatory arrest laws."[2] So it is no surprise that VAWA has had no discernible effect on intimate partner homicides over the last two decades.[3]

2. VAWA-funded programs have brought about widespread civil rights violations, including problems with sex discrimination,[4] denial of due process, and disregard of the presumption of innocence.[5]

3. VAWA programs are weakening the traditional family. Loose definitions of domestic violence allow for state intervention into even a heated argument or minor couple conflict. That intervention typically forces the partners to separate, escalates the conflict, and discourages reconciliation. In the end, children often end up in a single parent household, placing them at far greater risk of child abuse and other social pathologies.[6]

Problem	Explanation
1. VAWA programs have been ineffective in reducing partner abuse, and in some ways, have placed victims at greater risk of violence.	*Treatment of Abusers:* Many jurisdictions in the United States mandate abuser treatment programs based on the Duluth Model that have consistently been shown to be ineffective and disallow treatment based on sound science.[1,2] In many states, persons who conduct batterer intervention programs have no mental health training or qualifications.[3] Furthermore, few VAWA-funded services are available to help abusive women.[4] *Restraining Orders:* Research reveals that restraining orders are generally ineffective in preventing future physical violence.[5,6,7] One study found that protection order statutes were associated with an *increase* in the number of black women killed by their unmarried partners.[8] There is substantial doubt whether restraining orders do anything more than lull victims into a false sense of security.[9] *Mandatory Arrest:* Mandatory arrest laws were implemented as a result of VAWA 2000. Even though mandatory arrest was removed from the 2005 version of VAWA, such laws are still on the books in 23 states.[10] A recent analysis from Harvard University shows that mandatory arrest laws actually *increase* intimate partner homicides by 60%.[11] Thirty-three states have laws that impose mandatory arrest for violation of a restraining order, leading to arrests of persons for sending their children a birthday card and similar actions.[12] One study concluded that prosecuting violations of restraining orders was "associated with *increases* in the homicide of white married intimates, black unmarried intimates, and white unmarried females."[13]

Problem	Explanation
	Following the introduction of mandatory arrest laws, the number of 911 calls for domestic violence dropped by about 15%,[14,15] suggesting that mandatory arrest deters requests for police assistance.
	Human Trafficking:
	VAWA has been ineffective in stopping partner violence partly because it has become involved in issues that have nothing to do with partner abuse. For example, VAWA contains numerous references to human trafficking.
	Trafficking involves holding someone in the *workplace* through force, fraud, and coercion.[16] But domestic violence involves felony or misdemeanor crimes of *violence* between *intimate partners.* Linking the two issues confuses and weakens the effort to stop domestic violence.
2. VAWA undermines basic notions of civil liberties and the presumption of innocence.	*Definitions of Domestic Violence:* Civil law definitions of DV are so broad and evidentiary standards are so weak that any verbal dispute or disagreement between partners can be construed as domestic "violence" and becomes the grounds to issue a restraining order.[17]
	False Allegations: False allegations of domestic violence have become widespread.[18] In some cases, women who are involved in an extra-marital affair falsely accuse their husband of abuse once he discovers the affair.[19]
	Primary Aggressor Policies: Primary aggressor arrest policies and prohibitions on dual arrest promote gender profiling: "there is a growing effort to avoid arresting female *perpetrators* under a policy of arresting the 'primary offender'"[20] and "police may be adopting a more lenient attitude toward females."[21]
3. VAWA programs have had a disproportionate negative effect on minority and low-income populations.	*Mandatory Arrests:* Mandatory arrests have had a disproportionate effect on African Americans, who now represent 23% of all arrests between spouses and 35% of arrests between boyfriends/girlfriends.[22] The Ms. Foundation for Women notes, "Criminalization of social problems has led to mass incarceration of men, especially young men of color, decimating marginalized communities."[23]
	Legal Aid: Free legal services are available to alleged victims, but not to alleged offenders. Lower-income persons accused of domestic violence have little or no ability to find legal services. These persons are often forced to agree to an allegation for an offense they did not commit. Only 4% of recipients of VAWA-funded Legal Assistance for Victims services are male.[24]

Problem	Explanation
4. VAWA undermines the family, escalates partner conflict, and discourages reconciliation.	DV intervention programs typically do not distinguish between a one-time couple disagreement and severe physical violence; thus intrusive DV programs serve to escalate minor partner conflict. The safest place for men and women is in the intact family.[25] DV programs should seek to support the intact family whenever possible.[26] But VAWA-funded program policies[27] and state laws[28] actually discourage/prohibit couple counseling and mediation.
5. VAWA fosters sex-based discrimination.	The Omnibus Crime Control and Safe Streets Act of 1968, as amended, prohibits discrimination on the basis of sex. In 2005 Congress added the following requirement to VAWA: "Nothing in this title shall be construed to prohibit male victims of domestic violence, dating violence, sexual assault, and stalking from receiving benefits and services under this title."[29]
	Despite this provision, the DoJ continues to employ discriminatory language in its grant program titles (e.g., "Grants to Reduce Violence Crimes Against Women on Campus" and grant solicitations (e.g., "entities engaged in violence against *women* activities").[30] As a result, male victims continue to be subjected to widespread discrimination.[31]
6. VAWA promotes half-truths, myths, and falsehoods about domestic violence.	*Findings:* Most of the findings in the VAWA law are one-sided, misleading, or false.
	Training and Education: VAWA-funded training and education programs often lack balance and factual accuracy, routinely depicting men as aggressors and women as victims. That bias is so widespread that it is believed to be undermining civil liberties and prejudicing the even-handed administration of justice.[32]
	National Institute of Justice Evaluations: Most domestic violence evaluations conducted by the DoJ National Institute of Justice substantially downplay, or ignore altogether, male victims of domestic violence.[33] That violates congressional intent, and also violates 28 CFR 46.111(3), which requires DoJ-funded research to assure "equitable" selection of research subjects.[34]
7. VAWA encourages immigration fraud.	*Immigration:* VAWA amends the Immigration and Nationality Act so illegal aliens can obtain permanent residency, work permits, and U.S. citizenship from the Citizenship and Immigration Service by making an accusation of domestic violence, even if the allegation is unsubstantiated.[35,36] VAWA guarantees free legal services to immigrants who make a claim of abuse. In effect, this gives a strong legal advantage to an illegal immigrant over a U.S. citizen.[37]

Problem	Explanation
	VAWA confidentiality provisions preclude the ability of a U.S citizen falsely accused of domestic violence to present exculpatory evidence to immigration authorities or to present evidence of immigration fraud committed by a person who "self-petitions" the CIS.
	International Dating Organizations:
	The International Marriage Brokers Regulation Act (Sections 831-834 of VAWA) requires that international match-making organizations collect extensive criminal background information for every prospective client. This assumes that all clients of these agencies represent a threat to foreign nationals, and represents a violation of the notion of "innocent until proven guilty."[38]
8. VAWA programs lack accountability and allow wasteful use of taxpayer dollars.	Auditors have documented a long-standing pattern of financial mismanagement of VAWA-funded programs.
	The Government Accountability Office has repeatedly documented shortcomings in program oversight by the OVW, including "inconsistent documentation and the lack of systematic data,"[39]
	poor quality evaluations that "raise concerns about whether the evaluations will produce definitive results,"[40] and lack of program utilization data that would be "consistent and reliable enough for analysis of the specific information required."[41]
	Likewise the DoJ Office of the Inspector General has documented wide-scale financial mismanagement, both by recipients of OVW grants[42,43,44] and by the Office on Violence Against Women itself.[45] More than a year after the irregularities were identified, the problems remained unresolved.[46]
	Finally, reports have been received of embezzlement of VAWA funds[47] and falsification of federal financial reports.[48]

[1] D. Dutton, *The Abusive Personality: Violence and Control in Intimate Relationships* (New York: Guilford Press, 1998).

[2] L. Feder and D. B. Wilson, "A Meta-analytic Review of Court-mandated Batterer Interventions Programs: Can Courts Affect Abusers' Behaviors?" *Journal of Experimental Criminology* 1 (2005): 239–262.

[3] R. Maiuro and J. Eberle, "State Standards for Domestic Violence Perpetrator Treatment: Current Status, Trends, and Recommendations," *Violence and Victims,* 2006.

[4] Respecting Accuracy in Domestic Abuse Reporting, *Has VAWA Delivered on Its Promises to Women?* (Rockville, MD: RADAR, 2007), http://www.mediaradar.org/docs/VAWA-Has-It-Delivered-on-Its-Promises-to-Women.pdf.

[5] J. Grau, J. Fagan, and S. Wexler, "Restraining Orders for Battered Women: Issues of Access and Efficacy," *Women and Politics* 4 (1984): 13–28.

[6] A. Harrell and B. Smith, "Effects of Restraining Orders on Domestic Violence Victims," in *Do Arrests and Restraining Orders Work?* ed. C. Buzawa and E. Buzawa (Thousand Oaks, CA: Sage, 1996), 229.

[7] J. McFarlane, A. Malecha, J. Gist, et al., "Protection Orders and Intimate Partner Violence: An 18-month Study of 150 Black, Hispanic, and White Women," *American Journal of Public Health* 94, no. 4 (2004): 613–618.

[8] L. Dugan, D. Nagin, and R. Rosenfeld, *Exposure Reduction or Backlash? The Effects of Domestic Violence Resources on Intimate Partner Homicide,* NCJ Number 186194 (Washington, DC: National Criminal Justice Reference Service, 2001), http://www.ncjrs.gov/app/Publications/Abstract.aspx?ID=186193.

[9] Independent Women's Forum, *Domestic Violence: An In-Depth Analysis* (Washington, DC: IWF, 2005), http://www.iwf.org/specialreports/specrpt_detail.asp?ArticleID=815.

[10] N. Miller, *What Does Research and Evaluation Say about Domestic Violence Laws? A Compendium of Justice System Laws and Related Research Assessments* (Alexandria, VA: Institute for Law and Justice, 2005), http://www.ilj.org/publications/dv/DomesticViolenceLegislationEvaluation.pdf.

[11] R. Iyengar, *Does the Certainty of Arrest Reduce Domestic Violence? Evidence from Mandatory and Recommended Arrest Laws* (Cambridge, MA: National Bureau of Economic Research, June 2007).

[12] Respecting Accuracy in Domestic Abuse Reporting, *Justice Denied: Arrest Policies for Domestic Violence* (Rockville, MD: RADAR, 2006), http://www.mediaradar.org/docs/Justice-Denied-DV-Arrest-Policies.pdf.

[13] Dugan, Nagin, and Rosenfeld, "Exposure Reduction or Backlash?"

[14] L. Dugan, "Domestic Violence Legislation: Exploring Its Impact on the Likelihood of Domestic Violence, Police Intervention and Arrest," *Criminology and Public Policy* 2 (2003): 283–312.

[15] C. E. Corry, *Principal Effect of 1994 DV Law in Colorado Springs Is Reduction in 911 Domestic Disturbance Calls to Police* (Colorado Springs, CO: Equal Justice Foundation, 2001–2005), http://www.dvmen.org/dv-110.htm.

[16] Markon J. Human, "Trafficking Not Big U.S. Issue," *Washington Post,* September 23, 2007, http://www.washingtonpost.com/wp-dyn/content/article/2007/09/22/AR2007092201401_pf.html.

[17] Respecting Accuracy in Domestic Abuse Reporting, *Without Restraint: The Use and Abuse of Domestic Restraining Orders* (Rockville, MD: RADAR, 2006), http://www.mediaradar.org/docs/VAWA-Restraining-Orders.pdf.

[18] Respecting Accuracy in Domestic Abuse Reporting, *A Culture of False Allegations: How VAWA Harms Families and Children* (Rockville, MD: RADAR, 2007), http://www.mediaradar.org/docs/VAWA-A-Culture-of-False-Allegations.pdf.

[19] C. E. Corry, *Condoning Slavery under Color of Law* (Equal Justice Foundation, 2004), http://www.ejfi.org/family/family-74.htm, Colorado Springs, CO.

[20] M. A. Straus, "Future Research on Gender Symmetry in Physical Assaults on Partners," *Violence against Women* 12, no. 11 (2006): 1093.

[21] D. Hirschel et al., "Explaining the Prevalence, Context, and Consequences of Dual Arrest in Intimate Partner Cases," (April 2007, Washington D.C.): 170. www.ncjrs.gov/pdffiles1/nij/grants/218355.pdf.

[22] M. R. Durose, *Family Violence Statistics* (Washington, DC: Federal Bureau of Investigation, June 2005), NCJ 207846, Table 5.9.

[23] Ms. Foundation for Women, *Safety and Justice for All* (New York: Ms. FW, 2003), 17.

[24] General Accountability Office, *Services Provided to Victims of Domestic Violence, Sexual Assault, Dating Violence, and Stalking,* GAO-07-846R (Washington, DC: GAO, July 19, 2007), 24, www.gao.gov/new.items/d07846r.pdf.

[25] S. Catalano, *Intimate Partner Violence in the United States* (Washington, DC: U.S. Department of Justice, 2006), http://www.ojp.usdoj.gov/bjs/intimate/table/wommar.htm.

[26] National Family Violence Legislative Resource Center, *Policy Statement on Family Violence* (NFVLRC), http://www.nfvlrc.org/docs/NFVLRC_2_.Policy.statement.pdf, Sacramento, CA, 2008.

[27] J. Austin and J. Dankwort, "Standards for Batterer Programs," *Journal of Interpersonal Violence* 14, no. 2 (1999): 152–168.

[28] R. Maiuro et al., "Are Current State Standards for Domestic Violence Perpetrator Treatment

Adequately Informed by Research?" *Journal of Aggression, Maltreatment, and Trauma* 5 (2001): 21–44.

[29] Violence Against Women and Department of Justice Reauthorization Act of 2005, Section 40002(b)(8).

[30] For example, see FY 2007 Grants to State Sexual Assault and Domestic Violence Coalitions Program, http://www.usdoj.gov/ovw/docs/statecoalitions2007.pdf.

[31] Respecting Accuracy in Domestic Abuse Reporting, *VAWA Programs Discriminate against Male Victims* (Rockville, MD: RADAR, 2006), http://www.mediaradar.org/docs/VAWA-Discriminates-Against-Males.pdf.

[32] Respecting Accuracy in Domestic Abuse Reporting, *Education for Injustice* (Rockville, MD: RADAR, 2007), http://www.mediaradar.org/docs/.

[33] General Accounting Office, *Justice Impact Evaluations: One Byrne Evaluation Was Rigorous; All Reviewed Violence Against Women Office Evaluations Were Problematic,* Report No. GAO-02-309 (Washington, DC: GAO, March 2002).

[34] Protection of Human Subjects, *28 Code of Federal Regulations Part 46,* http://a257.g. akamaitech.net/7/257/2422/12feb20041500/edocket.access.gpo.gov/cfr_2004/julqtr/28cfr46.111.htm.

[35] J. Mann, *Beware Illegal Alien Women! (and Men),* August 4, 2003, http://www.vdare.com/Mann/illlegal_alien_women.htm.

[36] C. Roberts, *How Female Illegals Abuse the System,* ifeminists.net, September 13, 2007, http://www.ifeminists.net/e107_plugins/content/content.php?content.221.

[37] C. Roberts, *VAWA Gives More Rights to Illegals Than Citizens,* ifeminists.net, September 20, 2007, http://www.ifeminists.net/e107_plugins/content/content.php?content.226.

[38] W. McElroy, *Mail Order Bride Law Brands U.S. Men as Abusers,* ifeminists.net, January 11, 2006, http://www.ifeminists.net/introduction/editorials/.

[39] General Accounting Office, *Justice Discretionary Grants: Byrne Program and Violence Against Women Office Grant Monitoring Should Be Better Documented,* Report GAO-02-25 (Washington, DC: GAO, November 2001).

[40] General Accounting Office, *Justice Impact Evaluations.*

[41] General Accountability Office, *Services Provided to Victims of Domestic Violence.*

[42] Office on Violence Against Women, *Legal Assistance for Victims Grant No. 1998-WL-VX-0023, Legal Aid of Nebraska, Omaha,* Audit Report No. GR-60-05-012 (Washington, DC: DOJ, September 2005).

[43] U.S. Department of Justice, *Stop Violence Against Women Formula Grant Awarded to the State of Texas, Office of the Governor, Criminal Justice Division,* Audit Report No. GR-80-05-008 (Washington, DC: DOJ, August 2005).

[44] U.S. Department of Justice, *Grants to Encourage Arrest Policies and Enforcement of Protection Orders Administered by Dane County, Wisconsin,* Audit Report No. GR-50-04-003 (Washington, DC: DOJ, December 2003).

[45] U.S. Department of Justice, Office of the Inspector General, *The Department of Justice's Grant Closeout Process,* Audit Report 07-05 (Washington, DC: DOJ, 2006), http://www.usdoj.gov/oig/reports/plus/a0705/final.pdf.

[46] U. S. Department of Justice, *Management Decisions on Audit Reports Not Implemented within One Year, as of March 31, 2007* (Washington, DC: DOJ, 2007), http://www.usdoj.gov/jmd/alo/may2007/delinquent_audit_reports.pdf.

[47] "Theft Alleged at Abuse Shelter," *Pioneer Press,* St. Paul, MN, Feb.15, 2006, P. B-1.

[48] *SafeHouse Plans Last Appeal of $483,000 Penalty by State,* June 3, 2006, http://www.mlive.com.

NOTES

1. Respecting Accuracy in Domestic Abuse Reporting, *Why Have Domestic Violence Programs Failed to Stop Partner Abuse?* (Rockville, MD: RADAR, 2007), http://

www.mediaradar.org/docs/RADARreport-Why-DV-Programs-Fail-to-Stop-Abuse.
pdf (Accessed, October 22, 2007).

2. R. Iyengar, *Does the Certainty of Arrest Reduce Domestic Violence? Evidence from Mandatory and Recommended Arrest Laws* (Cambridge, MA: National Bureau of Economic Research, p. 3, June 2007).

3. S. Catalano, *Intimate Partner Violence in the United States* (Washington, DC: U.S. Department of Justice, 2006), http://www.ojp.usdoj.gov/bjs/intimate/ipv.htm (accessed, October 18, 2007).

4. Respecting Accuracy in Domestic Abuse Reporting, *VAWA Programs Discriminate against Male Victims* (Rockville, MD: RADAR, 2006), http://www.mediaradar.org/docs/VAWA-Discriminates-Against-Males.pdf.

5. Respecting Accuracy in Domestic Abuse Reporting, *Without Restraint: The Use and Abuse of Domestic Restraining Orders* (Rockville, MD: RADAR, 2006), http://www.mediaradar.org/docs/VAWA-Restraining-Orders.pdf.

6. Respecting Accuracy in Domestic Abuse Reporting, *A Culture of False Allegations: How VAWA Harms Families and Children* (Rockville, MD: RADAR, 2007), http://www.mediaradar.org/docs/VAWA-A-Culture-of-False-Allegations.pdf.

Notes

CHAPTER 1: IS IT REAL?

1. M. Straus and R. Gelles, "Societal Change and Change in Family Violence from 1975 to 1985 as Revealed by Two National Surveys," *Journal of Marriage and the Family* 48 (August 1986): 467. See also M. Straus, R. J. Gelles, and S. Steinmetz, *Behind Closed Doors: Violence in the American Family* (Garden City, NY: Anchor Press/ Doubleday, 1980), 20–22.

2. M. McLeod, "Women against Men: An Examination of Domestic Violence Based on an Analysis of Official Data and National Victimization Data," *Justice Quarterly* 1 (1984): 171–193.

3. J. A. Byles, "Family Violence: Some Facts and Gaps: A Statistical Overview," in *Domestic Violence: Issues and Dynamics,* ed. V. D'Oyley (Toronto: Ontario Institute for Studies in Education, 1978). See also Evaluation of Domestic Violence in the San Diego Region (1981), San Diego Association of Governments; and B. E. Vanfossen, "Intersexual Violence in Monroe County, New York," *Victimology* 4 (1979): 299–305, all cited in McLeod, "Women against Men."

4. U.S. Department of Justice, Bureau of Justice Statistics, http://www.ojp. usdoj.gov/bjs/intimate/report.htm (2007).

5. U.S. Department of Justice, Office of Justice Programs, *Violence against Women: Estimates from the Redesigned Survey,* Bureau of Justice Statistics NCJ-154348 (Washington, DC: Government Printing Office, 1995). See also idem, *Violence against Women: A National Crime Victimization Survey Report,* Bureau of Justice Statistics NCJ-145325 (Washington, DC: Government Printing Office, 1994), 6, 101.

6. McLeod, "Women against Men," 173.

7. Ibid.

8. G. M. Wilt, J. D. Bannon, R. K. Breedlove, J. W. Kennish, D. M. Sandker, and R. K. Sawtell, *Domestic Violence and the Police: Studies in Detroit and Kansas City* (Washington, DC: Police Foundation, 1977); cited in McLeod, "Women against Men."

9. U.S. Department of Justice, Office of Justice Programs, *Highlights from 20 Years of Surveying Crime Victims: The National Crime Victimization Survey, 1973–92*, Bureau of Justice Statistics NCJ-144525 (Washington, DC: Government Printing Office, 1993), 321.

10. W. Goldberg and M. Tomlanovich, "Domestic Violence Victims in the Emergency Department," *Journal of the American Medical Association* 251, no. 24 (June 22–29, 1984): 3259–3264.

11. Ibid., 3263. Because there were 275 females and 217 males in the total sample, 58 fewer men filled out the questionnaire. Thirty-eight men from this total said they were victims of domestic violence, while 62 women said they were victims. Given the smaller number of men available to respond, the authors did not find this difference in number to be "statistically significant." The authors also stated in the same paragraph: "Previous studies that suggest there may be a substantial number of male domestic violence victims have come under attack, not so much for their methodology as for their potential harm to the development of programs to aid women victims."

12. U.S. Department of Justice, *Violence-Related Injuries Treated in Hospital Emergency Departments,* http://www.ojp.usdoj.gov/bjs/ BJS98054 (1997).

13. D. Martin, *Battered Wives* (New York: Pocket Books, 1976/1983), 53–54.

14. Peter H. Neidig, "Executive Summary Family Advocacy Prevention/Survey Project Update: Overview and Preliminary Findings" (unpublished paper prepared for the U.S. Army by Behavioral Science Associates, Stony Brook, NY, 1993), 3.

15. Ibid.

16. R. L. McNeely and G. Robinson-Simpson, "The Truth about Domestic Violence: A Falsely Framed Issue," *Social Work* (November–December 1987): 485–490.

17. J. Giles-Sims, *Wife Battering: A Systems Theory Approach* (New York: Guilford Press, 1983), 50.

18. C. A. Hornung, B. C. McCullough, and T. Sugimoto, "Status Relationships in Marriage: Risk Factors in Spouse Abuse," *Journal of Marriage and the Family* 43 (1981): 675–692; cited by M. Straus in "Physical Assaults by Wives: A Major Social Problem," in *Current Controversies on Family Violence*, ed. R. J. Gelles and D. R. Loseke (Newbury Park, CA: Sage, 1993).

19. D. Thomas, *Not Guilty: The Case in Defense of Men* (New York: William Morrow, 1993), 186–187. Thomas is quoting Erin Pizzey, the founder of Chiswick Women's Refuge in England, the world's first battered women's shelter.

20. Martin, *Battered Wives,* xi.

21. These results from the National Family Violence Survey have been published many times in a number of publications. Further information can be obtained from these main sources: Straus and Gelles, "Societal Change," 465–479; M. Straus, "Sociological Research and Social Policy: The Case of Family Violence," *Sociological Forum* 7, no. 2 (1992): 212–237; and J. E. Stets and M. Straus, *Physical*

Violence in American Families: Risk Factors and Adaptations to Violence in 8,145 Families (New Brunswick, NJ: Transaction Press, 1990). The phrase "selective inattention" is from Straus, in "Physical Assaults by Wives: A Major Social Problem," in *Current Controversies on Family Violence,* ed. R. J. Gelles and D. R. Loseke (Newbury Park, CA: Sage, 1993). This may be the best single article on the methodology and context of various family violence studies, and its reference list is very complete. An interesting and fairly rare longitudinal (the same people across time) study is available by request to Rena. Sommer, "Male and Female Perpetrated Partner Abuse: Testing a Diathesis-Stress Model" (The Ph.D., dissertation at the University of Manitoba, Canada may not have been published as quoted here from her 1994 paper). The author states, "Even though we found a certain degree of recanting of abuse, the pattern of reporting remained the same. We also found that when respondents were asked to report on abuse during the past year, there was no significant difference between the males (7.1%) and females (6.6%) reporting." Also see the Selected Resources for an Internet address that provides a list of available literature related to domestic violence, including literature about male and female victimization.

22. L. Nisonoff and I. Bitman, "Spouse Abuse: Incidence and Relationship to Selected Demographic Variables," *Victimology* 4 (1979): 134, 137, 138.

23. Straus and Gelles, "Societal Change," 470.

24. Straus, "Physical Assaults by Wives," 69.

25. E. Lupri, "Harmonie und Aggression: Uber die Dialektick Ehlicher Gewalt (Hidden in the Home: The Dialectics of Conjugal Violence—the Case Canada)," *Kolner Zeitschrift fur Soziologie und Sozialphychologie* 42, no. 3 (1990): 5, 479–501. Because I do not read German, Dr. Lupri furnished me with the English translation of this paper, page numbers refer to this version, available from the University of Calgary, Department of Sociology, Alberta, Canada.

26. Ibid., 7, 11, 13.

27. Ibid., 8.

28. Ibid., 5.

29. P. Tjaden and N. Thoennes, "Extent, Nature and Consequences of Intimate Partner Violence: Findings from the *National Violence Against Women Survey*" (NCJ 181867) (Washington, DC: U.S. Department of Justice, Office of Justice Pro grams, 2000).

30. Daniel J. Whitaker, Tadesse Haileyesus, Monica Swahn, and Linda S. Saltz-man. "Differences in Frequency of Violence and Reported Injury between Relationships with Reciprocal and Nonreciprocal Intimate Partner Violence," *American Journal of Public Health* 97, no. 5 (May 2007): 941–947.

31. Straus, "Physical Assaults by Wives," 74.

32. Ibid., 75. See also L. D. Brush, "Violent Acts and Injurious Outcomes in Married Couples: Methodological Issues in the National Survey of Families and Households," *Gender and Society* 4 (1980): 56–57, for similar results from a national survey not conducted by Straus/Gelles and the Family Research Laboratory. See also note 21.

33. McNeely and Robinson-Simpson, "Truth about Domestic Violence," 486.

34. Amazon.com posted book review for this volume, posted June 16, 2001.

35. L. A. Gregorash, "Family Violence: An Exploratory Study of Men Who Have Been Abused by Their Wives" (master's thesis, University of Calgary, Alberta, Canada, 1993), 44.

36. McLeod, "Women against Men," 185.

37. Gregrorash, "Family Violence," 52.

38. McLeod, "Women against Men," 185.

39. Ibid.

40. Ibid., 185–186. Here McLeod cites M. Wolfgang, *Patterns in Criminal Homicide* (Philadelphia: University of Pennsylvania, 1975); and L. A. Curtis, *Criminal Violence* (Lexington, MA: D. C. Heath, 1974).

41. Ibid.

42. M. Straus, letter to author, 1995.

43. B. Morse, "Beyond the Conflict Tactics Scale: Assessing Gender Differences in Partner Violence," *Violence and Victims* 10, no. 4 (1995): 257–272.

44. R. L. McNeely, interview with author, October, 1995.

45. Gregorash, "Family Violence," 65.

46. J. Malone, A. Tryree, and K. O'Leary, "Generalization and Containment: Different Effects of Past Aggression for Wives and Husbands," *Journal of Marriage and the Family* 51 (1989): 690. See also Straus and Gelles, "Societal Change," 471, table; and K. O'Leary, J. Barling, I. Aria, A. Rosebaum, J. Malone, and A. Tyree, "Prevalence and Stability of Physical Aggression between Spouses: A Longitudinal Analysis," *Journal of Consulting and Clinical Psychology* 57, no. 2 (1989): 263–268.

47. The incident was reported in G. Sheey, *Hillary's Choice,* (New York: Ballantine Books, 2000) a generally admiring biography; in the Drudge Report; and in C. Anderson, *Bill and Hillary* (New York: William Morrow, 1999).

48. U.S. Department of Justice, Office of Justice Programs, *Murder in Families,* Bureau of Justice Statistics Special Report NCJ-143498 (Washington, DC: Government Printing Office, 1984).

49. K. Van Wormer, Amazon.com review of this volume, posted June 16, 2001.

50. DOJ, *Murder in Families.*

51. U.S. Department of Justice, Office of Justice Programs, *Survey of State Prison Inmates, 1991: Women in Prison,* Bureau of Justice Statistics Special Report NCJ-145321 (Washington, DC: Government Printing Office, 1994), 3.

52. C., Mann, "Getting Even? Women Who Kill in Domestic Encounters," *Justice Quarterly* 5, no.1 (1988): 33–50.

53. Ibid., 48–49.

54. C. McCormick, *Battered Women: The Last Report* (Chicago: Cook County, Department of Corrections, 1976).

55. C. Mann, interview with author, 1994.

56. *Survey of State Prison Inmates,* 4.

57. S. Steinmetz, interview with author, 1994.

58. Gregorash, "Family Violence," 39.

59. Straus, Gelles, and Steinmetz, *Behind Closed Doors,* 100–101.

60. Ibid., 101.

61. N. O'Keefe, K. Brockopp, and E. Chew, "Teen Dating Violence," *Social Work* (November–December 1986): 465–468.

62. C. Forsyth, G. Wooddell, R. Evans, "Predicting Symmetry in Female/Male Crime Rates," *Journal of Police and Criminal Psychology* 16, no. 2 (Fall 2001): 1–9.

63. Straus, "Physical Assaults by Wives," 79.

64. McNeely and Robinson-Simpson, "Truth about Domestic Violence," 487.

65. S. Steinmetz, "The Battered Husband Syndrome," *Victimology* 2 (1977): 499.

66. Gregorash, "Family Violence," 89.

67. L. Miller, "Violent Families and the Rhetoric of Harmony," *British Journal of Sociology* 41, no. 2 (1990): 61–286; cited by E. Lupri, in "Spousal Violence: Wife Abuse across the Life Course," *Kolner Zeitschrift fur Soziologie und Sozialphychologie* 13 (1993): 232–257.

68. Steinmetz, "The Battered Husband Syndrome," 499.

69. Martin, *Battered Wives,* 30.

70. M. Brinkerhoff, E. Grandin, and E. Lupri, "Religious Involvement and Spousal Abuse: The Canadian Case," *Journal for the Scientific Study of Religion* 31, no. 1 (1992): 15–31. *Note:* Refer to the bibliography by Fiebert at the University of California–Long Beach for further studies since 1992, which replicated these results in the United States.

71. K. Lobel, ed., *Naming the Violence: Speaking Out about Lesbian Battering* (Seattle: Seal Press, 1986), 98–102. See also C. M. Renzetti, *Violent Betrayal: Partner Abuse in Lesbian Relationships* (Newbury Park, CA: Sage, 1992).

72. Renzetti, *Violent Betrayal.* See also Lie and Gentlewarrior, "Intimate Violence in Lesbian Relationships," *Journal of Social Science Research* 15 (1987): 41–59; and C. Card "Lesbian Battering," *Newsletter on Feminism and Philosophy* (November 1988): 3.

73. A. Frodi, J. Macaulay, and P. Ropert-Thome, "Are Women Always Less Aggressive Than Men? A Review of the Experimental Literature," *Psychological Bulletin* 84, no. 4 (1977): 634–654.

74. W. Farrell, *The Myth of Male Power: Why Men Are the Disposable Sex* (New York: Simon and Schuster, 1993), 283. Cited in Elizabeth Brookin's observational study of adolescents at El Camino High School, Oceanside, CA, 1989–1992.

75. *Esquire,* February 1994, 65.

76. N. Angier, *New York Times* News Service, June 1995, reporting on the proceedings of the Endocrine Society.

77. T. Lewin, *New York Times* News Service, May 1992.

78. David Crary, AP National Writer, Associated Press, New York, June 16–17, 2001.

CHAPTER 2: TELLING THEIR STORIES

1. L. A. Gregorash, "Family Violence: An Exploratory Study of Men Who Have Been Abused by Their Wives" (master's thesis, University of Calgary, Alberta, Canada, 1993), 89; M. J. George, "A Preliminary Investigation of Instrumental Domestic

Abuse of Men," *Memorandum 14 to the Home Affairs Committee* (Department of Physiology, Queen Mary and Westfield College, London, 1992); C. Engbritson, interview with author, February 1996.

2. M. Straus and R. Gelles, "Societal Change and Change in Family Violence from 1975 to 1985 as Revealed by Two National Surveys," *Journal of Marriage and the Family* 48 (August 1986): 471.

3. M. J. George, interview with author, March, 1996.

4. *The Oregonian,* April 17, 1993, A1, A18; August 17, 1993, C1, C14.

5. Nancy Bein, executive producer of CBS-TV movie *Men Don't Tell* (1993), interview with author, June, 1996.

6. G. Saenger, "Male and Female Relations in the American Comic Strips," *The Funnies: An American Idiom,* ed. D. M. White and R. H. Abel (Glencoe, NY: Free Press, 1963), 219–231.

7. Sylvia Ashton, as quoted by M. J. George, in an interview with the author, June, 1996.

8. R. Johnston, attorney, interview with author, July, 1996.

CHAPTER 3: THE DOMESTIC VIOLENCE TRAP

1. G. Hankins, *Prescription for Anger: Coping with Angry Feelings and Angry People* (New York: Warner, 1993), 17–18.

2. R. L. McNeely, and G. Robinson-Simpson, "The Truth about Domestic Violence: A Falsely Framed Issue," *Social Work* (November–December 1987): 488.

3. M. Straus, R. J. Gelles, and S. Steinmetz, *Behind Closed Doors: Violence in the American Family* (Garden City, NY: Anchor Press/Doubleday, 1980), 141.

4. Ibid., 140.

5. Ibid., 150.

6. Ibid., 148.

7. J. Sherven, and J. Sniechowski, interview with author, October, 1996.

8. Straus, Gelles, and Steinmetz, *Behind Closed Doors,* 141.

9. Interview with author, October, 1996.

CHAPTER 4: RESISTANCE AND ACCEPTANCE

1. S. Steinmetz, "The Battered Husband Syndrome," *Victimolgoy* 2 (1977): 507.

2. S. Steinmetz, interview with author, February, 1994.

3. E. Pleck, J. Pleck, M. Grossman, and P. Bart, "Comment and Reply: The Battered Data Syndrome: A Comment on Steinmetz Article," *Victimology* 2, nos. 3–4 (1977–1978): 680–684.

4. S. Steinmetz, "Reply to Pleck, Pleck, Grossman and Bart," *Victimology* 2, nos. 3–4 (1977–1978): 683–684.

5. S. Steinmetz, interview with author, 1994.

6. D. Lees, "The War against Men," *Toronto Life* (December 1992): 104.

7. M. Straus, "Physical Assaults by Wives: A Major Social Problem," in *Current Controversies on Family Violence,* ed. R. J. Gelles and D. R. Loseke (Newbury Park, CA: Sage, 1993), 67–87.

8. R. L. McNeely, interview with author, 1994.

9. R. L. McNeely and G. Robinson-Simpson, "The Truth about Domestic Violence: A Falsely Framed Issue," *Social Work* (November–December 1987): 485–490.

10. Murray Straus, "From Ideology to Inclusion: Evidence-Based Policy and Intervention in Domestic Violence" (paper presented at the National Family Violence Legislative Resource Center conference, Sacramento, CA, February 15–16, 2008). Material Used by permission and somewhat modified in format here. Donald Dutton, Ph.D., also presented similar examples in this regard at the same conference.

11. C. A. Hornung, B. C. McCollough, and T. Sugimoto, "Status Relationships in Marriage: Risk Factors in Spouse Abuse," *Journal of Marriage and the Family* 43 (1981): 675–692. Cited by Straus, "Physical Assaults by Wives," 67–87.

12. E. G., Krug, L. L., Dahlberg, J. A., Mercy, A. B., Zwi, and R. Lozano, *World Report on Violence and Health.* Geneva: World Health Organization, 2002.

13. D. Thomas, *Not Guilty: The Case in Defense of Men* (New York: William Morrow, 1993), 185–191.

14. Lees, "The War against Men," 104–106.

15. C. H. Sommers, "Figuring Out Feminism," *National Review* (June 27, 1994): 30–34.

16. J. Hallinan, Newhouse News Service, July 7, 1994.

17. Donna E. Shalala, Secretary of Health and Human Services, American Medical Association's National Conference on Family Violence, Washington, DC, March 11, 1994.

18. U.S. Department of Justice, *Violence-Related Injuries Treated in Hospital Emergency Departments,* http://www.ojp.usdoj.gov/bjs/ BJS98054 (1997).

19. Proclamation 7129—National Domestic Violence Awareness Month, 1998: September 30, 1998—Pres. Bill Clinton—Transcript: By the President of the United States of America:

A Proclamation: Domestic violence is a leading cause of injury to American women, and teenage girls between the ages of 16 and 19 experience one of the highest rates of such violence. A woman is battered every 15 seconds in the Untied States, and 30 percent of female murder victims are killed by current or former partners. Equally disturbing is the impact of domestic violence on children. Witnessing such violence has a devastating emotional effect on children, and between 50 and 70 percent of men who abuse their female partners abuse their children as well. From inner cities to rural communities, domestic violence affects individuals of every age, culture, class, gender, race, and religion.

The actual radio address to the nation by President Clinton used slightly different language and used a different set of statistics, such as "every 12 seconds."

"In America today, domestic violence is the number one health risk for women between the ages of 15 and 44. Close to a third of all women murdered in this country were killed by their husbands, former husbands or boyfriends. Every 12 seconds, another woman is beaten. That's nearly 900,000 victims every year.

And statistics tell us that in half the families where a spouse is beaten, the children are beaten too. Domestic violence is a criminal activity. It devastates its victims and affects us all. It increases health costs, keeps people from showing up to work, prevents them from performing at their best. It destroys families, relationships and lives, and it tears at the fabric of who we are as a people."

20. J. Griffith, "Husband Survives the Lumps and Bumper of a New Marriage," *The Oregonian,* September 21, 1993.

21. J. Griffith, interview with author, 1994.

22. M. George, interview with author, 1994.

23. W. Cronkite, speech to Radio Television News Directors Association Convention, Las Vegas, NV, 1979.

24. M. Straus and G. Kaufman-Kantor, "Cultural Norms Approving Marital Violence: Changes from 1968 to 1992 in Relation to Gender, Class, Cohort, and Other Social Characteristics" (unpublished report, Family Research Laboratory, University of New Hampshire, Durham, 1994).

25. N. Bein, interview with author, 1994.

26. J. Light, interview with author, 1994.

27. M. Thomas, interview with author, 1994.

28. M. Hess, interview with author, 1994.

29. G. Gilliand, interview with author, 1994.

CHAPTER 5: EXPLORING NEW APPROACHES TO REDUCING DOMESTIC VIOLENCE

1. L. Sherman, "Domestic Violence," in *National Institute of Justice Crime File Study Guide,* NCJ-97720 (Washington, DC: Government Printing Office, 1985). This publication makes note of a Police Foundation study that found the following: "The official records showed that about 18 percent of all offenders repeated their violence, while only 10 percent of the arrested offenders repeated it."

2. Portions of this chapter appeared in *Family Interventions in Domestic Violence: A Handbook of Gender-Inclusive Theory and Treatment,* ed. J. Hamel and T. Nicholls (New York: Springer, 2007), 601–619. Coauthors of the article were Cathy Young, Philip W. Cook, Sheila Smith, Jack Turtletaub, and Lonnie Hazelwood. Used by permission. Portions also appeared in Cathy Young, "Domestic Violence and In-Depth Analysis," September, 2005, posted on Independent Women's Forum Web site, http://www.IWF.org.

3. L. Mills, *Insult to Injury: Rethinking Our Responses to Intimate Abuse* (Princeton, NJ: Princeton University Press, 2003).

4. Ibid.

5. See D. N. Heleniak, "The New Star Chamber: The New Jersey Family Court and the Prevention of Domestic Violence Act," *Rutgers Law Review* 57, no. 3 (2005): 1009–1042. Also see: Suk, Jeannie, "Criminal Law Comes Home," *The Yale Law Journal*-116:2 (2006), http://www.yalelawjournal.org/pdf/116-1/Suk.pdf. Accessed October 12, 2008. Some relevant quotes from this document include: "Through prosecutors' routine deployment of protection orders in the criminal process at arraignment, plea bargaining, and sentencing, the home is becoming a space in which criminal law deliberately reorders and controls private rights and relationships in property and marriage—not as an incident of prosecution but as its goal. The growing criminal law use of protection orders to prohibit the cohabitation and contact of intimate partners (often when substantial jail time is not imposed) is a form of state-imposed de facto divorce that subjects the practical and substantive continuation of intimate relationships to criminal sanction." p. 2. And, "The expanding definition of violence, mandatory arrest, no-drop policies, the prosecution of many more cases than can ultimately be proven, and the decreasing emphasis on imprisonment are all developments that contribute to making de facto divorce a de facto solution to DV. As de facto divorce becomes a more prevalent alternative to traditional punishment, it is likely to reinforce the expansion of the definition of DV crime and an increase in DV arrests and prosecutions for nonviolent conduct, as law enforcement personnel increasingly imagine the consequences of bringing such domestic incidents into the criminal system to be less draconian than incarceration. A wide range of nonviolent conduct in the domestic space then becomes subject to criminal law regulation, down to the existence of an intimate relationship itself. What becomes visible is a shift in emphasis from the goal of punishing violence to state control of intimate relationships in the home. This shift is not completely accomplished, but it is underway." p. 70.

6. See Los Angeles Gay and Lesbian Center, http://laglc.convio.net/site/Page Server?pagename=homepage.

7. M. Hofford and A. Harell, "Family Violence Interventions for the Justice System," in *Program Brief, Bureau of Justice Assistance,* NCJ-144532 (Washington, DC: Government Printing Office, 1995), 19. This source notes, "The failure of judges to respond appropriately in family violence cases was cited as the biggest single problem faced in the majority of the demonstration projects."

8. K. Van Wormer and S. Bednar, "Working with Male Batterers: A Restorative-Strengths Perspective," *Families in Society: The Journal of Contemporary Human Services* 83, no. 5 (2002): 557–565.

9. E. Pence, *Coordinating Community Responses to Domestic Violence: Lessons from Duluth and Beyond* (Thousand Oaks, CA: Sage, 1999), 25–40.

10. J. Austin and J. Dankwort, "A Review of Standards for Batterer Intervention Programs," *Violence Against Women Online Resources,* www.biscmi.org/other_resources/docs/massachusetts.html (accessed August 3, 2002).

11. Commonwealth of Massachusetts Executive Office of Health and Human Service, Department of Public Health, *Massachusetts Guidelines and Standards for the Cer-*

tification of Batterers' Intervention Programs, www.biscmi.org/other_resources/docs/
massachusetts.html (accessed March 5 1995).

12. (1) ORS 180.700 gives the Attorney General authority, in consultation with
an advisory committee, to adopt rules that establish standards for batterers intervention programs (BIP). OAR 137–087–0000 through 137–087–0100 establish
those BIP standards for intervention services provided to male batterers who engage in battering against women, http://arcweb.sos.state.or.us/rules/OARS_100/
OAR_137/137_087.html (Adopted January 1, 2006. Accessed February 5, 2006).

13. Pence, *Coordinating Community Responses,* 25–40.

14. L. Meckler, Associated Press wire service report, January 1, 1996. The source
citied here is Jim Zepp of the Justice Research and Statistics Association in a survey
conducted for the U.S. Department of Justice.

15. U.S. Census Bureau, http://www.census.gov/Press-Release/www/releases/
archives/income_wealth/012528.html.

16. J. Dimmitt, interview with author, March, 1994.

17. L. Menand, "The War of All against All," *The New Yorker,* March 14, 1994, 85.

18. Woods. v. Shewry; 3rd Dist. C056072 http://www.courtinfo.ca.gov/opin
ions/documents/C056072.PDF.

19. A. Trice, A. Huges, C. Odom, K. Woods, and N. McClellan, "The Origins of
Children's Career Aspirations: IV. Testing Hypotheses from Four Theories," *Career
Development Quarterly* 43, no. 4 (1995): 307–322. These authors state, "Girls aspired
to higher level jobs than boys at every grade level" (315). They also reported: "Boys
were twice as likely as girls to mention sex-inappropriateness as a reason for reject-
ing a job.... These findings, taken in conjunction with previous studies, might suggest either that male stereotyped jobs have become more accessible to girls than
female-stereotyped jobs have become accessible to boys, either through changes
in the nature of the workplace or because deliberate efforts have been undertaken
to make traditionally men's jobs more inviting to girls, whereas fewer efforts have
been made to make traditionally women's jobs inviting to boys" (319).

20. G. Botvin, E. Baker, L. Dusenbury, E. Botvin, and T. Diaz, "Long-Term
Follow-up Results of a Randomized Drug-Abuse Prevention Trial in a White
Middle-Class Population," *Journal of the American Medical Association* 273, no. 14
(1995): 1106–1112. Copies of the Life Skills Training Program are available through
Princeton Health Press, Inc.; for information, call: (609) 921–0540.

21. E. Daggy, interview with author, April, 1994.

22. L. A. Gregorash, "Family Violence: An Exploratory Study of Men Who Have
Been Abused by Their Wives" (master's thesis, University of Calgary, Alberta, Canada, 1993), 102–103.

Selected Bibliography

Cose, Ellis. *A Man's World: How Real Is Male Privilege—and How High Is Its Price?* New York: HarperCollins, 1995.

Farrell, Warren. *The Myth of Male Power: Why Men Are the Disposable Sex.* New York: Simon and Schuster, 1993.

Giles-Sims, Jean. *Wife Battering: A Systems Theory Approach.* New York: Guilford Press, 1983.

Hamel, John. *Gender-Inclusive Treatment of Intimate Partner Abuse: A Comprehensive Approach.* New York: Springer, 2005.

Hamel, John, and Tonia Nicholls. *Family Interventions in Domestic Violence.* New York: Springer, 2007.

Kammer, Jack. *Good Will toward Men: Women Talk Candidly about the Balance of Power between the Sexes.* New York: St. Martin's Press, 1994.

Kline, James. *The Whole Truth about Domestic Violence.* Dillon, CO: Swan Mountain Press, 2003.

Lobel, Kerry, ed. *Naming the Violence: Speaking Out about Lesbian Battering.* Seattle: Seal Press, 1986.

Martin, Del. *Battered Wives.* New York: Pocket Books, 1983.

Pearson, Patricia. *When She Was Bad: Violent Women and the Myth of Innocence.* New York: Viking, 1997.

Pizzey, Erin, and Jeff Shapiro. *Prone to Violence.* London: Hamlyn Paperbacks, 1982.

Solomon, Rob. *Full Esteem Ahead: Keys to Strong Personal Values and Positive Self-esteem.* Newport Beach, CA: Kincaid House, 1992.

Sommers, Christina Hoff. *Who Stole Feminism? How Women Have Betrayed Women.* New York: Simon and Schuster, 1994.

Straus, Murray, Richard J. Gelles, and Suzanne K. Steinmetz. *Behind Closed Doors: Violence in the American Family.* Garden City, NY: Anchor Press/Doubleday, 1980.

Thomas, David. *Not Guilty: The Case in Defense of Men.* New York: William Morrow, 1993.

Young, Cathy. *Ceasefire! Why Woman and Men Must Join Forces to Achieve True Equality.* New York: Free Press, 1999.

FURTHER READING

Cook, Philip W. "Female Violence against Men Is a Serious Problem." In *Domestic Violence,* ed. Tamara Roleff. San Diego: Greenhaven Press, 2000.

Cook, Philip W. "The Whole Truth about Domestic Violence." In *Everything You Know Is Wrong,* ed. Russ Kick. New York: Disinformation Press, 2002.

McNeely, R. L., and Philip W. Cook. "Notes on Newspaper Accounts of Male Elder Abuse." *Journal of Elder Abuse and Neglect* 19, nos. 1/2: 99–108 (2007).

McNeely, R. L., Philip W. Cook, and Jose Torres. "Violence as Seen through a Prism of Color. Part II: Is Domestic Violence a Gender Issue, or a Human Issue?" *Journal of Human Behavior in the Social Environment* 4, no. 4: 227–251 (2001).

Selected Resources

Abused Men: www.abusedmen.com. My personal Web site. Members of the news media and those interested in contacting me for speaking engagements should contact me through this site. Because of volume, I cannot respond to personal requests for help. The site does contain links to some helping organizations. Additional helping organizations and those organizations with a keen interest or primary focus on the issue are listed here.

Annotated Bibliography of Domestic Violence Research, California State University, Long Beach, Martin Fiebert, Ph.D.: http://www.csulb.edu/~mfiebert/assault.htm

Domestic Abuse Helpline For Men and Women: www.dahmw.info/1–888–743–5754.

Independent Women's Forum: http://www.iwf.org/ifeminists.com: http://www.ifeminists.net

Family Non Violence: http://www.familynonviolence.org/National Coalition of Free Men: http://www.ncfm.org/

National Family Violence Legislative Resource Center: www.nfvlrc.org

Respecting Accuracy in Domestic Abuse Reporting (RADAR): http://www.mediaradar.org/

Stop Abuse For Everyone: http://www.safe4all.org/

True Equality Network: http://true-equality.org/

Index

About the Author

PHILIP W. COOK is an investigative journalist who has won numerous awards from the Associated Press and the Society of Professional Journalists. He has appeared in interviews on CNN, MSNBC, Fox Network's *The O'Reilly Factor,* and been heard on 75 radio talk shows nationwide. He has also been quoted by the Associated Press and 40 daily newspapers across the United States, Canada, and Great Britain. Before becoming a journalist, he was Executive Director of the PACE Institute for Families in Transition in Portland, Oregon.